Yogini's Dilemma

Yogini's Dilemma

*To Be, or Not to Be,
a Yoga Teacher*

NICOLE A. GRANT
CERTIFIED YOGA THERAPIST

NEW YORK

LONDON • NASHVILLE • MELBOURNE • VANCOUVER

Yogini's Dilemma
To Be, or Not to Be, a Yoga Teacher

© 2020 NICOLE A. GRANT

Published in New York, New York, by Morgan James Publishing in partnership with Difference Press. Morgan James is a trademark of Morgan James, LLC. www.MorganJamesPublishing.com

ISBN 978-1-64279-774-9 paperback
ISBN 978-1-64279-775-6 eBook
ISBN 978-1-64279-776-3 audio
Library of Congress Control Number: 2019914194

Cover Design by:
Megan Whitney
megan@creativeninjadesigns.com

Interior Design by:
Bonnie Bushman
The Whole Caboodle Graphic Design

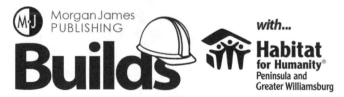

Morgan James is a proud partner of Habitat for Humanity Peninsula and Greater Williamsburg. Partners in building since 2006.

Get involved today! Visit
www.MorganJamesBuilds.com

To my father,
Who shone the light on basic human decency.

Yoginis,
There are four sources of life energy, or prana:

Breathing—so breathe, in and out, wide and deep.
Food—eat to nourish your body and soul.
Environment—nurture it.
And True Self, the gift of You—how will you manifest this in the world?

To bring the essence of You into Action in the world is Teaching Yoga.
Herein unfolds the path…

Table of Contents

Preface

Winchester, MA—April 8, 2019

I believe I found yoga, or yoga found me, because of the person my father was in the world and who I wanted to be in his image. When he passed away, there was so little room in my life to grieve. And so it was that a little over two years after his passing, at thirty-six, I found myself trekking in the Himalayas. The draw was the Valley of Flowers, a rare high-altitude Indian valley that, at 11,500 ft (3,505 m), has long been acknowledged by renowned mountaineers and botanists as one of the world's most richly diverse natural botanical gardens.

It was a leap of utter faith but the call to meet myself in a spiritual setting as far away from my grief was that great. There was a brief overnight in Rishikesh, located in the foothills of this Himalayan mountain range in northern India. Rishikesh is known as the Gateway to the Garhwal Himalayas because of its scenic seat on the Ganges River where it flows down from the mountains. While Rishikesh is a magnet for spiritual seekers and is, now more than ever, the Yoga

Capital of the World, the sheer congestion of humanity overwhelmed me so completely.

And so, I found myself on my first steep climb stretching to 14 km from Gauri Kund to Kedarnath, a small, stone village nestled within the awesome majesty of the surrounding mountains and pastures, at a height of 11,755 ft (3,583 m) above sea level. Kedarnath Temple, one of Hinduism's holiest shrines dedicated to Lord Shiva, (one of the Hindu trinity of gods) stood out in the otherwise barren and unattractive township. Seven years later, it would survive bearing the brunt of nature's fury in the massive flash floods of 2013 that swept through Uttarakhand. Back in August of 2006, it was here that I suffered my first ever panic attack. I was halfway around the world, in thin air, having left my children behind with my mother and their father, freaking out that I would succumb to altitude sickness or get bitten by a rat that one of my co-trekkers had come across in her bunk, or, worse yet, die in a landslide. Landslides are a common occurrence in this area, more so with the building of dams in this violently active geologic zone. In the midst of panic, I heard the sound of my own voice soothing me, *Breathe in, breathe out. Count your breath Nicole…Slower, louder, make it longer, deeper, breathe in-one-breathe out, breathe in-two-breathe out…*

I made it to the next morning, rather worse for wear, and through the next days. Then on to Badrinath and Badrinath Temple, another Hindu temple, this one dedicated to another god of the Hindu trinity, Vishnu, the Perseverer, my kind of guy. There, in the dark of night, in the middle of nowhere, I heard the spine-chilling rumble of my first Himalayan landslide. I held my breath and prayed, *Please let me see my children again. Please. Please. I will live my life according to my own truth. Please let me hold my family.* It is astounding what truths reveal themselves in one's awareness when death comes calling. I had to acknowledge it wasn't just my father I was grieving, but the failings of my marriage too. I was in relationship to someone who wasn't the person I thought he was; or perhaps, he simply wasn't the person I wanted him to be. *You weren't there for me when my father died, when I needed you most. You hurt my heart with your deceptions. I don't know how to trust you anymore.* As the mountain shuddered and heaved, I curled up into a very small ball, praying for my life, praying to be with my loved ones, praying to find myself, in truth, again.

These mountains taught me what letting go (of the things I was holding onto) feels like and what faith is. I learned to surrender to these rhythms of nature beyond my control, for the simple fact I had no choice but to do so. These experiences paved for me a different, more authentic way of being in the world. I found my feet as the morning mist spilled out in front of me, navigating the rocky and alternating ascendant and descendant paths and river crossing to the spectacular Valley of Flowers. Known as Bhyundar, the valley is a womb-filled basket of flowers, abound with Purple Asters, rose-petalled lady slipper Cypripedium, pink geraniums, dwarf irises and indigo-colored Nomocharis, white and red potentillas and so many more, each species blooming and flowering according to their own calendar.

This trek was a respite from the fearsome travels by bus along the one-lane Himalayan mountain roads. As we were transported from one destination to another, we would stop sometimes for hours at a stretch while a landslide here or there was cleared away. I would gaze out at the distant Nanda Devi and then zoom in on a bird sitting on a phone wire to stay focused in the moment. I was sitting on the side of the bus that overlooked the deep gorge of nothingness beyond the missing road's edge; looking down was not an option.

I don't care for heights. And yet, trek the Himalayas I did. I believe it is this journey I took to the farthest reaches of my world that brought me right up against my greatest fears but also showed me how to dig deep for strength I did not know I had. I had not intended to make the noble trek to one last spiritual destination—Hemkund Sahib, a clear water lake at 14,300 feet—but something within me felt compelled to make this pilgrimage of the Sikhs. You cannot stay overnight here due to the too-rapid exposure to low amounts of oxygen at high elevation. I cannot say if it was a mild symptom of acute mountain sickness or an adrenaline rush from the dauntingly steep climb or maybe this confrontation with the great unknown, but during my sojourn of thirty minutes at the far side of the lake amongst the stark beauty and bounty of brahma kamal, large, white, lotus-like flowers, I felt the soft tug of heartstrings and the warm embrace of my departed father. With the gentle echo of voices of Sikh men dipping in the frigid waters wafting through an impenetrable curtain of fog, I laid my father's spirit to rest.

My father, bless his spirit, knew me better than I knew myself. He always asked the right questions at the right time, and I gave the answers I wanted to believe according to a false understanding of what I thought I wanted in life at that time. I was twenty-six when I became engaged and my father asked me, "Will you have enough space for yourself in this relationship?" I didn't think twice about considering what his question was actually asking but simply responded, "Of course. I know I will be happy enough. I love him." And it's not that I didn't. It's just that, back then, I was looking outside of myself to feel complete, at this relationship for a sense of worthiness and lovability, and at marriage for something that felt safe and 'known'. And my father knew it.

When my father passed away, I had been married for just over seven years, and I had two beautiful, healthy, wholesome children, ages two and a half and six. We had an unusual and wonderful home in a lovely town, and I was the proud, albeit overwhelmed and unsupported-by-my-spouse co-owner of a sweet little yoga studio. Nothing about running the 'business' came easy to me, but it allowed me the flexibility in my schedule to raise my children and do something I was passionate about. I was teaching a lot of yoga just to keep the studio doors open, and feeling very insecure about doing so as I never felt 'good enough'. At that time, it was customary for the yoga practitioner to receive the blessing of her teacher in order to pursue teaching yoga. I would receive this validation a few years later from my Ashtanga teacher, Nancy Gilgoff, but meanwhile thrust myself into teaching with vigor and passion having participated in an informal yet substantial pre-Yoga Alliance ashtanga vinyasa yoga training with Beryl Bender Birch and Thom Birch. When I reflect on this time, I imagine my husband must have thought I was having a love affair with my yoga, given the energy and time I devoted to it. From my perspective, I got to do something that I loved AND made me a better person; it freed me too from a commute that kept me away from home and family for too many hours of the day given the extent to which my husband traveled. And yet, I remember thinking to myself, *Is this all there is to my life?* I felt the lack within myself and perhaps in my partner as well, and as habit would have it, went looking outside myself to fill the hollow.

And so, this is how I found myself, at thirty-six, trekking in the Garhwal Himalayas. I didn't know it at the time, but my yoga was slowly opening me up to my Self. I held onto a good number of things—like my paradigm of family and the life I thought I wanted for myself— afraid to sever myself from all that was 'known' and more afraid still to walk alone. It turns out, I'm a baby-steps kind of person, or was. Little by little, step by step, breath by breath, I began traveling in the direction of my heart's calling. Please know, it was not at all clear to me at the time what that looked like, where I was headed or even what I was doing. But what did happen is I began to build the confidence I needed to trust myself.

Over the years, all the stuff that felt 'not-right' in my life started falling away. The discomfort or hurt I suffered was all relative to how hard I held on to the very things I thought I needed. I lived a cultural dynamic of seeking solutions to problems that aren't real, or trying to fix or manage or control the problems that are; I felt the need to accomplish and attain goals I didn't actually want for myself; and my actions served to gratify the whims and desires of a mind driven by a lack of clear intentionality and sense of Self. It turns out that, while it is very possible to create yourself in the image of who you [think you] want to be in your mind, it is harder to live it if it does not align with who you actually are. It is in getting to know your mind that you turn towards your Self and say, *Ah, there you are my sweet Self! How I have forgotten you. I wish to return to you and know you deeply.* In working with your yoga to figure out who (or where) you are, you become more and more the you *You* were always meant to be.

This book is written as a series of letters to You, dear yogini, who have extended me the privilege at some point or another, or still, of serving as your guide on your yoga journey; to You who are traveling the path of yoga and picked up this book because you got curious; and to my younger self too—the far more naïve me who got detoured by the current of her life and then happened upon this well-worn path of practice over two decades ago at a time of need.

In my travels, I have discovered an immense wealth of common sense and discernment in yoga and meditation and extend my deepest gratitude to those teachers I met along the way who have walked this path before me and shared with me the wisdom of their own experiences. If there is one thing I take away from my long-term study of this art and science, it is that it is indeed a practice. There are no magic bullets or spontaneous solutions to the problems of life and living—even though I still catch myself seeking them out at inopportune moments. But there is magic, and it lives in the unfolding of the yogic process, this shining of the diamond in the rough to reveal its innate brilliance.

As I persevere at living my life with awareness and in the full spectrum of my humanness, I see the resistances that show up in my body and in my monkey-mind more and more for what they are. Then I notice how they show up in my life as well. What am I fighting against in my body? In my thoughts? In my soul? What am I choosing to fight in my life? Who am I entering into conflict with if not with some aspect of myself? What feels purposeful and what does not? Did I always want to be a yoga teacher, or do I teach yoga because of some mysterious unfolding of life and living?

Ask yourself, dear yogini, what is driving your question: *To be or not to be a yoga teacher?* Are you incentivized by how much your yoga practice has changed you in your personal life, and perhaps you truly seek to extend to others the wisdom and benefits of your own experiences? Are you in it to make a life change and want to learn more about the methodology of yoga and Yogic Wisdom? Is it your perceived solution to a problem you think you have? What kind of practitioner of yoga are you, and what kind of teacher would you be? I urge you to pose yourself these questions in practice and rest into the answers. It is a worthwhile effort to use your yoga to understand what motivates your inquiry, for it is more likely than not, not the actual question you seek an answer to. Yet, a training program that guides you with care and attends to your asking can serve you to optimal effect.

We are each a reflection of one another's humanity. If you picked up this book, there is a strong possibility that yoga is the equation you are working with to live into the answers to any number of questions, with this one as your focal point perhaps. I have discovered that there are usually far more questions than there are answers and that living life with intentionality and sincerity of heart is the more favorable path to receiving an honest and frank response. Our collective attempts to resolve our questions and manipulate their outcome to meet the ideals in our head reveal the resistances within ourselves. So pay close attention to the body in *āsana* and the mind in meditation as you take your seat in practice. You have a special gift to offer, of this I am sure; allow your yoga to reveal this to you so you may then transport this out into the world as an agent of change, yoga teacher or not.

This is the path of yoga. Pay close attention to all that shows up in your awareness, those sneaky implicit biases and conditioned ways of looking out upon the world for they are the sources of our discontent and suffering. Self-preoccupation, it turns out, is not the same as self-awareness. This is my personal motivation for getting to know my mind better, if not to reduce my own torments, then perhaps to minimize their effects on others. While pleasing everyone is not an option, living in harmony with oneself and those you choose to surround yourself with is. My sincere hope is that our combined practices will ripple out into the world with the effect of supplanting the negativity and disconnect so prevalent today with positivity, community and connection.

May you persevere in your practice with audacity and heart.
May you be filled with loving kindness.
May you be well and safe.
May you be happy and free.

In friendship and support,
Nicole

PROLOGUE

Excerpts From
My Personal Journal

Cambridge, MA—Wednesday, June 22, 1994

Today is not a good day. My mom called from Switzerland with not so great news: The big C word. My initial reaction was an overwhelming feeling of panic. It's weird how everything just goes blank for that split second that feels like an absolute eternity; I remember hearing the raucous palpitations of my heart, not to mention how it felt like it might explode out of my chest. Then I remember my mom asking me if I was still there. Yep. "I'm here," I say, although that's a bare truth indeed, given the way my mind is reeling (freaking out really). As I write this, my mind is spinning with all the unsolicited information which, because of my state of being at the time, comes back to me in mere fragments right now: Non-Hodgkin's lymphoma, T-cell, aggressive, caught early— 'They' think—small red mark on the bridge of her nose—that was what sent her to the doctor in the first place. This feels so surreal. It's not really happening. Is it? Is this what shock feels like? I am sitting with this news now, pen in hand, thinking I must do something. What can I do? My mind is grasping for straws, desperate for a solution to this problem that is an ocean away. I feel small and pitiful and useless and sad and…So many tears falling onto these now wet pages…

Cambridge, MA—Tuesday, June 28, 1994

This has got to stop. My stomach has been churning since I got my mom's call. I feel so anxious and agitated. I figured I'd get a massage or something to make me feel better and ended up receiving 'polarity massage'. I don't really know what that means, and the woman talked me into taking her yoga class—which was insane! Who knew yoga could be this…I can't really describe it but wow! I feel… Alive.

Geneva, Switzerland—Thursday, August 4, 1994

I've been here for almost three weeks now, helping Mom through her first chemo treatment. I gave up two part-time jobs to get the time off to fly home, so now I have just the one at the American Red Cross which I'm hoping will turn into something more. I nearly had a heart attack when I got off the plane in Geneva to see her waiting for me on the other side of the glass windows, nothing but skin and bone. The fortnight it took for her diagnosis to come back (positive) was when she lost all the weight, she says, from the worrying. I am beginning to realize how much I have taken my super-small world for granted. On top of that, it's gone topsy-turvy, a complete mishmash of contradictory thoughts and random beliefs that have no foundation in reality whatsoever—even I can see that. As of now, I feel untethered from the center of my own universe and am no longer here to serve just me; there's so much more at stake than I could have fathomed. I am so aware and freaked out by just how ephemeral life really is. And there is something going on with my health, I'm sure of it. I keep dreaming I have all these different types of cancer. Last night it was skin cancer; before that, breast cancer. At this point, I've diagnosed myself with pretty much every type of cancer I've ever heard of and know, at the deepest level of my being, that this torment doesn't lead anywhere worthwhile. Dad and I are up together in the wee hours of the morning, watching old movies on TV in nocturnal companionship (we watched a pirated and very poor-quality video of *Top Gun* last night and *Chariots of Fire* the night before), neither of us able to find sleep, scared of where our thoughts will take us. I don't know how my mother manages. The treatment sucks. I'm afraid of her dying and it's the first time I'm saying this 'out loud'. I know my Dad is scared stiff of the possibility of her dying too. I think it is that we find solace in our mutual fear. My unenthused imagination and mind games are driving me insane. I have to do something about this because the not-doing anything is of no help to me at all.

Cambridge, MA—Thursday, August 18, 1994

I feel it is some curious unfolding of the universe that has guided me straight into the rigorous yet comforting arms of Ashtanga Yoga. I'm not sure about the teacher though. She's making us memorize the sequence of the whole first series of postures, which is a solid 90-minute practice and complete anguish from start to finish; but I do love the way it wrings me out. I feel like I've come back to myself. It is so completely intense and textured with quasi-militaristic undertones, something to do with the count. For the most part, we don't sustain the poses for long periods of time and I like that! It offers me temporary respite from the nauseating rollercoaster ride of all these emotions I'm feeling and this mental trainwreck of mine. It's disciplined, and that's what I need right now. My practice is unceremonious at best, but all those years of ballet have given me a leg up in some respects. The downward-facing dog pose is killing me. My heels feel miles away from the floor, although thankfully I don't feel it too much in the backs of my legs. I'm practicing it every day in our downstairs gym now. My yoga mat is fast becoming my happy place.

Cambridge, MA—Thursday, January 5, 1995

I'm discovering a whole language in yoga that is really helping me frame and understand the stuff I'm experiencing; at the very least, I don't feel like my heart aches quite so much, and I don't have to deal with all the chatter in my head when I'm doing yoga. And besides, I'm killin' it! (This seems like an un-yogic sort of thing to say, but I'm quite accomplished at the yoga poses). All that German I had to study in high school is a real asset to learning the Sanskrit names of the postures—a lot of compound words and such, very cool. A tentative thought crossed my mind today, but I caught whiff of it so maybe it is meaningful: Maybe I could be a yoga teacher someday. I dunno, maybe not; I don't have enough experience, and the idea of it is giving me a panic attack already!

CHAPTER 1

Dilemma

*"The end of all our exploring will be to end where we started and
know the place for the first time."*
– T.S. Eliot

Winchester, MA—January 9, 2019

Dear Yogini,

You may have come to yoga by way of *asana*, the postural practice,
as I did, for reasons of sanity; or perhaps, as a way to address health
concerns, to meet fitness goals, to gain physical strength and flexibility.
Maybe it is that you needed space to breathe, to find release from the
stresses of life, to ground yourself in the physical body, to rediscover
community. Or maybe, like me, you stumbled into yoga out of sheer
necessity because another aspect of your life was falling apart at the

seams. And now, some time later, it has come to this: *Do I want to be a yoga teacher, or not?*

I so appreciate that you have sought me out with your question and trust. Know you are not alone in your quest for resolution. When you are short on time and low on inspiration the vicissitudes of life can feel overwhelming. You might be tempted to jump onto your yoga mat, or crash a class, and just go through the motions. Your mind, meanwhile, is seeking an answer to this question (or another that lies behind it), weaving its tales of worship or woe and all the reasons why you should become a yoga teacher and even better reasons why not to. By showing up for yoga, you plan to derive maximum value from your yoga with a physical practice, soothe the energies of emotions which have run amok, and quell your frazzled or, at best, distracted mind. And it figures, by practice's end, you have found a solution to a problem that's not yours and still remain baffled as to what on earth to do with your own quest for a satisfying outcome. You had a decent practice so maybe you can shelve the question for another day. Until it comes up again in your consciousness...

While the only direct experience I can speak to is mine, I do have an understanding of the struggles you face, the anxiety that undermines your best efforts, and your dilemma of whether to teach yoga or remain its faithful student (which you would continue to be regardless of the outcome of your decision). It is not within my purview to resolve anything about your life, but I am here in service of the courage you reveal in daring to show up for it.

I do wonder where the question of whether to teach or not comes from. Meanwhile, I invite you to persevere at your practice with diligence and to pay close attention to the stuff that comes up for you. Challenge yourself when you feel like begging off and keep showing up with your own particular brand of inner resolve so the yoga can guide you to where you want to be. We are our own best teacher. So, place your dilemma at your own feet and bow to your inner *guru*, dispeller of darkness. Teach yourself to be present for everything that shows up—the good and the bad, the hard and the soft, the strong and the weak, the joys and the sorrows—with humility and as much tenderness in your heart as you can fathom; if you are anything like me, you can be so hard on yourself. In those instances, notice that too.

First things first. You profess to have a dilemma in your heart, a situation in which you cannot decide whether to be a yoga teacher or not. Words, you will find, are of primordial importance to the yogin, avid practitioner of yoga, for they serve to qualify, describe, and discern your most intimate experiences of yourself. Whether you become a yoga teacher or not, the words you use to define your practical contact with a pose or an observation you make in the context of your yoga practice will have import and require more specificity as you make this journey.

The yogic teachings are so rich because they are imbued with the rich cultural heritage of India and the powerful language of yoga that is Sanskrit, which itself bears the meaning 'perfected' or 'refined' and is one of the oldest, if not the oldest, of all attested human languages. It behooves you then, dearest yogini, to dive into the dilemma your question poses.

If you consider the meaning of dilemma, it seems that 'dilemma' cannot be used to refer to something that is merely problematic. At its origin, dilemma referred to a choice between two equally unsatisfactory or unattainable options, or to an argument in which an opponent is given two options to choose from, neither of which is of particular service to the opponent. This is not necessarily your situation, but it could be. Have you never found yourself in conflict with yourself, and therefore in opposition to your best interests? I know I have. It's the proverbial rock and hard place. Who isn't in conflict with themselves about something or another? Do you ever wonder where that unsettled feeling of guilt comes from? You got it: *Dilemma*.

Dilemma would appear to refer to the state of mind that is marked by your uncertainty or doubt. It is not that you are faced with a classical dilemma, that choice between two equally unsuitable or unattainable options, because neither of your outcomes—to be a yoga teacher, or to not be a yoga teacher—is inherently unsuitable or unattainable. The unsuitability or unattainability of the options lies primarily in your mind. This feeling of entrapment—the 'either/or'—leads you down a path that limits your experience of the infinite possibilities and potential of *You*.

Travel with me, dear yogini. I do not claim to have mastered the path of yoga. Far from it. It is only that I am walking this mysterious path as my teachers have walked this path before me. I only pass on to you what I have discovered for myself along the way. It is for you to take what serves you in this moment and reject that which does not. If you receive a directive from me that does not make sense to your mind, that confuses or frustrates you, simply take notice. You always have the option to shelve it and revisit it at a more opportune time or discard it outright. If the lesson is important, it will cross your path again, at a time perhaps when you are ready to receive it. Of this, I have no doubt.

On some level, each of us participates in our own 'hero's journey' to remember who we are, what we are, and where we are on this path of life. You may have come to yoga with a slightly obsessive craving for *asana*—the practice of posture—or maybe you decided to try it out because it is said to help with stress and tension in the body. We tend to be consumers of yoga poses here in the West, but even if we shortchange ourselves with this incomplete form of yoga, it remains a valuable practice. Whether you are a mild practitioner or hardcore in your approach, if you do the yoga long enough, there is a pretty good chance you will see changes in your lifestyle or maybe even in the way you want to, or choose to, live your life; it is almost inevitable because somewhere along the path the yoga deepens our respect for life on every level.

Yoga originates from India and is based in rituals and sacrifice (of the ego). It seeks to explore the 'subject' (the mind) as a way of comprehending the outer world (science). While *Darshanas* are the philosophical and experiential systems of yoga, ways of 'seeing' the world, *The Yoga Sūtras of Patañjali* systematize the wisdom, or psychology, into a single text—the ultimate treatise of yoga that unifies the scattered and ancient Indian ritual practices and teachings of the Vedas. It offers a classical understanding of the mind and freedom from the ego-bound rigidity of the physical body, our energetic-emotional being and the mind. In Indian philosophy, our 'being-ness' is associated with neither the body nor the mind, as both can be controlled and exist externally to the innermost Self.

All yoga systems are designed to free the individual from habit patterns of mind, body, and speech to return to *atman*—the soul—in order to exist beyond the normal human condition. What makes yoga such a powerful practice is that we get to step outside of our habitual environment and relationships, the habitual happenings and doings of each day to see our habitual tendencies for what they are. While our place of practice is typically the mat or the cushion, our ultimate objective is to return to the place of practice that is our very own heart. This *bhava*, or 'becoming,' means that we return with mindful intent to who we already are.

Atha yogānuśāsanam, states the opening aphorism of Patañjali's manifest, *The Yoga Sūtras*: Here and now begins the discipline of yoga, of coming back into union with one's Self—our heroine's journey.

From this compilation of aphorisms attributed to the sage Patañjali from mid-second century BCE, we know him to have been an ascetic. Ascetics approach the world by turning away from it—the monks, the nuns, the renunciants, the *sadhus*. The Sanskrit scriptures describe the world as transitioning through cycles of four stages, each transition coinciding with rare planetary alignments. It is said we are in transition from the Kali Yuga—age of strife, discord, quarrel, or contention—to meet the age of truth, or Sat(ya) Yuga, by turning towards the world we live in and a humanity governed by intrinsic goodness. Is it possible that the world we are experiencing today is in fact a manifestation of darkness dissolving as we now begin to see reality—our collective ignorance and intelligence—for what it is?

Your decision to walk the path of yoga, dear yogini, emboldens you to engage with this momentum of consciousness rising that will serve someday soon to supplant the power-driven ego of today's world. Let us embrace ourselves in this spirit of truth. Persist in your efforts, dear yogini, and you will surely live into what you are looking for.

Sincerely,

Nicole

January 30, 2019

Dear Yogini,

Your dilemma is what leads the way. I practice yoga because the language of yoga speaks straight to my soul. Do you feel the same? Therefore, I shall speak to you of Patañjali. His manifesto lies at the foundation of all yoga in the West, and the path of yoga described in Chapter II (Book 2) of his *Yoga Sūtras* is the course we shall follow throughout these pages. Know that it serves as the framework to many 'Teacher Training' programs, although too many, in my humble opinion, shortchange the cultural heritage of yoga. The substance of yoga is steeped in its rich history, rituals and tradition, and our practice is powerful because of this.

So please indulge me and hear the story of Patañjali from the Puranas, a vast genre of Indian literature about a wide range of topics, particularly myths and legends, which illustrates only too well that the questions we pose and the dilemmas that embroil us in our mind don't always have clear-cut answers, or least not ones we might expect. Behind the stories lie fundamental truths, and sometimes, it isn't until the answer shows up that you realize the true question.

Once upon a time in the land of the Indo-Aryan subcontinent, the holy men and Rishis approached Lord Vishnu, the second god in the Hindu triumvirate (or trinity of gods known as *Trimurti*) responsible for the upkeep of the world, to tell him that even though he had proffered them the means to cure illnesses through Ayurveda, people still fell ill, and they wanted to understand what to do when sickness—not just physical ailments but such mental and emotional afflictions as anger, lust, greed, jealousy, desire, and pride—were manifested. Was there a formula to rid the beleaguered of their ailments and ease their suffering? Vishnu was lying on the coiled form of the serpent Adishésha with a thousand heads when the Rishis approached him. Upon their request, he gave them Adishésha, the symbol of awareness, who took birth in the world as Maharishi Patañjali.

Patañjali manifested on this earth to give us this knowledge of yoga which came to be known as the yoga sutras. The sage said he was not going to discuss the yoga sutras unless one thousand people gathered together. So, a thousand people gathered south of Vindhya Mountains to listen to him. Patañjali had one other condition: that a screen be placed to separate him from his students and that no one was to lift the screen or leave until he was finished with his teachings. Patañjali transmitted his knowledge to the thousand gathered from behind the curtain that concealed him. Each in attendance absorbed this knowledge, although they could not fathom how it was the Master was making each of them understand without uttering words. With wonderment, each experienced a shock of energy that was hard to contain, yet remained disciplined and attentive. One young enthusiast fell prey to nature's call and left the room thinking he might leave quietly and return as quietly so that his absence not be noticed. Another became curious and reflected, "I want to see the Master and what he is doing behind this curtain." He got so curious that he lifted the veil to look, but as he did so, all nine hundred and ninety-nine disciples were burned to ashes.

Patañjali became dejected to see that he had been ready to impart all knowledge to the whole world yet now had no disciples to carry forth the wisdom. In this moment, the one who had discretely left to seek out nature returned and asked forgiveness from Patañjali for his untimely departure. The great Master saw this as both an opportunity to retain at least one disciple to whom he could impart the rest of the yoga sutras and remaining knowledge whilst also teaching an important lesson. So Patañjali declared the young disciple a *Brahmarakshasa*, or (mythological) ghost, to be hanged on a tree. "To liberate yourself from this curse," instructed the sage, "you must teach one student the knowledge I have given you." And with this, Patañjali vanished.

Poor Brahmarakshasa hung from a tree for a thousand years, unable to find a single person to teach. Out of compassion, Patañjali returned disguised as Brahmarakshasa's one student to relieve the poor figure from the burden of the curse, and for seven days, from the top of the tree where the Brahmarakshasa hanged, he transliterated the sutras onto palm leaves. In a state of exhaustion, the sage set down the leaves near his garments and went to bathe, only to return to find a goat had eaten most of the leaves. Patañjali picked up what was left of the transliterations and walked away.

The story goes that to redeem one disciple, the Master became the disciple of a disciple. There is depth here and more questions than answers: *How does the Master convey knowledge to everybody without a single utterance? Why is the young disciple's absence of import? What is the significance of the veil? What is the message behind the Brahmarakshasa? What is the significance of the goat? What lessons does the story impart for you?* It is for the reader to unlock its meaning. And so, I leave you now, dear yogini, with these contemplations.

Sincerely,

Nicole

February 3, 2019

Dear Yogini,

The story of Patañjali tells us that yoga does not come with all the answers, and that life rarely unfolds according to plan. When I began my practice of yoga, I did so thinking it would somehow serve to mitigate the bad things in life from coming my way; that by engaging in this spiritual exercise of yoga, I could control outcomes and deflect negativity, meanness, and strife. It turns out, the yoga is simply there to help you pick yourself up when you fall and transmute perceived failures into productive feedback.

The gift of yoga is the way in which the persistent practice of it erodes the most steadfast stronghold of moral rectitude, softens, or categorically breaks open the hardest of hearts, and exposes the soft underbelly of uncertainty and fear that drives our loss of touch with reality. At first, you try too hard; you fight with feverish vigor, struggle with stubborn resistance to what is, to arrive at a particular posture, let's say, all the while striving for some idea of 'success' or feeling of 'accomplishment' that exists only in your mind. These ideals have the potential to drive you to greater heights—so long as your efforts remain intentional and sincere. They can also undermine your most valiant efforts when misguided and practiced without some degree of wisdom, leading to injury or dejection.

At some point you will see, if you have not yet, that yoga has the capacity to permeate every single layer of neurosis and reveal the objectionable nature of the stories the ego-brain tells. Over time, you will start to hear the voices in your head that do not belong to you and never have, the narratives you've adopted because you knew no better, and the dramas of your life that you have participated in that are not your own. Take your time learning this potent practice, for it has the richest of riches to share with you. Do not relinquish your inner resolve, for it will take you to some marvelous places!

February 10, 2019

Dear Yogini,

I perceive yoga's ultimate gift to be in that one breath that gives us pause so that we may notice the subtlest moments that are so ordinary and so simple that we miss them all the time: When you witness the first colored tint of sunrise on the horizon or, more evanescent still, the gentle expression on a stranger's face meant just for you that makes you smile because you are seen in that one split second you chose to lift your gaze from the constant companionship of the device in your hand. Maybe too, you've received the tender gift of that transient feeling of arriving in a pose and knowing its perfection in that one instant when ego, intellect and thoughts dissolve and you feel yourself a body of light.

Meanwhile, how do we stop listening to the internal stream of to-dos, how do we hit the pause button on the inner critic, how do we mitigate past hurts so they don't fragment this precious sphere of life? Are you able, and willing, to silence or step away from the buzz and rings and pings to be in your practice? Yoga is an alchemical practice, a way forward in experiencing yourself honestly, but only if you are wholehearted and tenacious in your willingness to engage the process.

Yoga is a way to get into the nitty gritty where your question abides: *To be, or not to be, a yoga teacher?* First, you will be directed to evaluate your attitude and practices towards others and then towards yourself. Mostly, though, you will be swayed by the physical realm— the ways in which your body is governed by habits and how it engages with movement, direction, and space. You will discover that there is nothing but distraction upon distraction—discomfort, aches and pains, frustrations at not understanding, irritation at not being able to 'do,' and myriad other discontents arising from your body and fomenting in your mind.

Your mind then becomes the object of your curiosity. At first, of course, when you start to perceive the persistent and inciting churnings of your thinking, you might believe yourself to be a little, or a lot, crazy around the edges. You can fall off the wagon here, take the other fork in the road, deviate from your very best intentions, say to yourself, *Not today. Not tomorrow. I do not have the patience for this. I'm not [fill-in-the-blank] enough.*

Excuses are a dime a dozen and impediments to your practice. I am the Queen of excuses, worst offender. So, yes, I will call you on yours because I am familiar with and can predict pretty much every single one you will come up with. The instant you perceive your excuse, your grievance or your resistance to whatever shows up in your sphere of awareness, whether it be physical, emotional, mental, intellectual, is the moment you begin your practice of yoga, *Atha yogānuśāsanam*. In my own self-study, I came across another expression of this sutra: "*Yoga (union) is the containment of one's ways of thought.* (1)" Learn this very first thread of wisdom from Patañjali's *Yoga Sūtras,* for it will come up again and again and again because you have chosen this path to answer your question.

The fact that you are engaged in this self-inquiry tells me three things about you:

1. You are a seeker.
2. You are already following the path of yoga whether you consider yourself to be a yogini or not.
3. You wish to know the direction of your travels.

You already know that the yogic path imparts wisdom beyond measure. I can only extend to you what I know from personal experience to be true of these yogic practices as applied to my own life. I hope to open and connect you to the very real magic of yoga, even though I can tell you that it does not always appear or feel magical in the moment. This means partaking in the hardships and the struggles that come up in the body and the mind, the impossible circumstances and unimaginable obstacles that appear as a function of life, and the complete and utter inevitability and vulnerability of being human.

I don't know how you came to yoga. It may be that your body weathered injury and you must be patient enough in your practice to seal the wound and make your own way 'home'. It may be that your life left you shipwrecked and stranded, and your yoga offers you a whole new way of existing in the world. Or you bailed out of necessity or by your own volition on some aspect of your life, leaving behind the known and knowable. Either way, you found yourself gazing out at the vast ocean of uncertainty before you. Maybe it still feels this way to you. As you continue to invite change into your life, there are always those around you who will feel threatened by your boldness and attempt to hold you back. It will feel like resistance until you are able to say, "I love you, and I must let you go." This is not to dissuade you from your course, dearest yogini; rather it's to encourage you to stay fierce and focused and true to yourself. No matter the circumstances, the not knowing what comes next is a fearsome and frightening feeling, and you will need all of your inner resolve to guide you.

It takes a remarkable kind of courage to travel this path of self-knowing, especially when you consider what you may be leaving behind. You might dip your toes in the water of yoga, or dive in out of some shade of desperation as I did to salvage myself from a marriage that was consuming too much of me. Sometimes you will have a choice in the matter; and maybe you will feel you have no choice at all. Whether you find yourself in shallow waters or deep you will learn that you already have within you the ability to wade and swim.

Herein rests the enchantment of yoga. It is the hint of the rosebud's color before its tint is discerned, or the scent of lilac before its fragrance is released into the air. It is the essence of the butterfly while still a caterpillar in the process of metamorphosis before emerging from the sanctum of her cocoon. The magic of yoga is in how it garners our full and undivided attention in the subtlest moments and with the simplest pleasure. You know all this of course. How then does it manifest in practice?

I hope to elucidate for you the wisdom of yoga that has been passed down through the ages as it pertains to your practice and to your life. On the one hand, it is up to the *sadhaka*, the spiritual aspirant, to follow this path of wisdom as a means to master herself. And on the other, it is the teacher's mission to shed light upon the path for the student rather than to promote her own self-mastery.

You will discover that your teacher was (and is still) a student like you, just as you will one day impart the teachings of yoga—as a teacher or not—with your own story to tell. You will learn that your teacher's achievements and successes are not there to be emulated or superseded. Rather, you will come to understand that your teacher's path has nothing to do with yours other than the fact that both of you are traveling as subjects of the human condition in search of your unique inner brilliance.

Be willing to explore beyond the surface level of platitudes and dive into the deepest, darkest, refracted places but only if it feels safe to do so in the moment. Learn to love yourself unconditionally regardless of anyone else's opinion of who you are or what you should (or should not) do. Get to know your mind, for a whole world of possibility will open to you as you step into the power of seeing things clearly as they are and reality as it is. Here and now, it is possible for you to experience yoga and realize your individual truth. The place to start is with who you already are, where you are right now, and what you are experiencing in this very moment. I have the benefit of my own experiences to illustrate for you how yoga works in life and thank you for allowing me to serve as your guide on this particular and powerful journey.

Peace and truth.

Warmly,

Nicole

CHAPTER 2

Daring to Be Me

"Yoga does not remove us from the reality or responsibilities of everyday life but rather places our feet firmly and resolutely in the practical ground of experience. We don't transcend our lives; we return to the life we left behind in the hopes of something better."
— **Donna Farhi**

February 14, 2019

Dear Yogini,

Hindsight, it turns out, offers a different reality than the one that is our present. There are tableaus from my life that reveal themselves to me now as irrefutable truths I could not claim to see then. I was too close to be able to focus on what needed to be seen, too blind to their inner workings, too young to do anything about it, too naïve to recognize a dynamic that was hurtful or cruel, too unwise or uncertain to change course. But I have sought my eternal verity for as long as I can remember. The Yogic Wisdom and practices have provided me with the tools to bridge the divide between my false cognition of reality, and the one that is reflected to me in truth.

At age seven, I made myself scarce, retreating to the beloved kingdom of my bedroom. There, my collection of dolls from far-off lands—each a gift from my father upon his return from mysterious travels to mysterious lands—transported me to a place of my own imagining. My bed with its yellow-and-white-plaid spread would call me in divine sleep where, instead of counting sheep, I would make up stories in my head to send me off into sweet slumber. There, I gazed out my bay windows from my nook at the color of rain spilling over the terrace and shrubs to pool at my new-planted acorn, soon to become an Oak. *Someday, when I am gone from here, I will be honored by this mighty presence.*

I lost myself in search of some understanding of something akin to God in the landscapes of Robert Frost and prayers to the divine. My mother appeared to not be inclined towards religion at all, and my father was a self-proclaimed atheist—though I have always doubted that, for he was far too adventurous by nature, a cat with nine lives in his lifetime, to not have had some faith in something. My home, as lovely as I remember it being, lacked in prayers of gratitude and blessings.

My first passion, besides the ethereal specter of God, was horseback riding. I have come to believe that perhaps it wasn't so much the riding of horses that I was most passionate about but rather that the horses saw me for who I am far more than I could see myself. I was a painfully shy child, so the truth of the matter is I had no need to be anyone other than myself around these intuitive creatures. My second romance was ballet, or classical dance which I pursued until I was nineteen. The rigor and discipline of the practice suited my personality. More than anything, I loved this embodied expression of how I felt. To this day, dance is still a direct path to my heart.

Dance fell by the wayside as I lost my sense of self to a curated idea of what I believed my life should be. I wanted to be a doctor, or so I thought. It turns out, my father hadn't the stomach to become a physician—he hated the sight of blood!—but wanted a medical professional of high standing in the family. And of course, I wanted to please my dad so I applied to medical school—three times (without fully committing to the process). During that period (of six years) my mother was diagnosed with T-cell non-Hodgkin's Lymphoma and I fell into yoga hard because of that diagnosis. On my mat I found respite from the churning of emotional turmoil and imagined outcomes around my mother's cancer. In yoga practice I stepped away from my weary attempts to get into medical school. Through yoga, I discovered a language that touched my soul.

In the face of my mother's disease, yoga offered me ground when everything else felt so fickle and ephemeral, each sun salutation a humble offering of my ego and a bow to the uncertainty of "what next?" Up until now, I had taken my life quite for granted without any conscious awareness of this. I just didn't know any better, this privilege of a 'me-myself-and-I' existence. Then my mother was declared 'in remission', marriage and children entered stage right, and life was great for a while.

My world contracted again as September 11, 2001 sent shockwaves of grief and anger through each and every heart. At this point I was teaching yoga full-time. I walked into my first post-9/11 yoga class, locking eyes with a yoga practitioner and friend who had been out of the country at the time. Nothing had to be said to know her life had been tragically impacted. I later learned her brother was missing. He worked in one of the towers and would never be found. A singular image of that tower faltering, floundering, and crashing is engraved as tautness and tears and darkness in my somatic memory. On the first anniversary of 9/11, my friend was in attendance at the memorial service at Ground Zero. She told me she saw the spirit of her brother in a multitude of dragonflies that seemed to embrace her. Years later, one early summer's day, I sat on a rock looking out over the crystalline blue of a reservoir, sort of meditating, being content. I became absorbed in a swarm of huge dragonflies flitting to and fro, right there in front of me. I was struck by their grandeur and the gossamer-like fabric of their wings reflecting the sun's brilliance, blinding diamond sparkles. I never carry my phone with me when I seek out nature for the purpose of being with myself for a while. But on this day I had, and the urge to reach out to my friend to let her know about the dragonflies was so compelling I texted her to say, *I am thinking of you my friend.* I'll never forget her reply: *Today is my brother's birthday.*

In almost every part of the world, the dragonfly symbolizes a transformative shift, adaptability and self-realization. This transformative shift has its source, says yoga, in mental and emotional clarity and maturity which in turn lends understanding to the deeper meaning of life. While I embrace the symbolism, the larger lesson is this: *Pay attention.* There is extraordinary eloquence in these ephemeral moments too easily missed because our focus is not-present.

The community yoga studio I co-founded with my friend Sarah Church opened up on the heels of 9/11. Those first years of the studio were turbulent as I navigated the newness of motherhood and the death of my beloved father who lived in Switzerland at the time. Have you ever looked back at a time in your life, dear yogini, and wondered how you made it through? This experience bred a certain fierceness in me that extended onto my mat and into my yoga. I would push through the moments that got hard and let anger steal my grief as I'd grind through my daily primary series practice, one posture superimposed upon another.

With my yoga, I have weathered the joys and sorrows of my life and navigated too dramatic changes in the yoga industry as a whole that reflect yoga's soaring popularity. My yoga studio and its community of yoga practitioners have been the one constant through all of it. My most heartfelt realization is that I have not done any of the hard stuff alone. I just kept showing up, one foot in front of the other, forward motion. In this community I found solace when I was in pain. In this practice I found ground beneath my feet. In the friends I have made through my yoga, I sought wisdom when I felt confused, or worthless, or insecure, or categorically insane. No time more than when I went through my divorce.

A family weekend getaway to Montreal as a surprise for my fortieth birthday—a Labor Day weekend—brought everything in my married relationship to a head. The weekend itself was fine at the level of platitudes, but I have never felt more alone, rejected, or deceived in my entire life. Kids asleep in their queen-sized bed, I joined my husband at the hotel bar in the lobby.

"What's going on?" I prompt. He is already onto his second or third drink, whatever it is. He is drowning any attempt at self-expression in alcohol. I am still stuck in benign non-understanding. All I feel is this huge disconnect between us, a massive ravine, and always his discomfort. He is slouched over the bar, squirming on his stool.

"I don't know," he says.

"What's with you and these events you have to travel to and projects you have to complete, on weekends, during planned holidays? And now, you want to leave Montreal early? It's my birthday and YOU brought me here… I need you to explain this to me. Are you having an affair with a woman at work? I need to know."

He shrugs his shoulders, "Have you seen the women I work with?"

What's that supposed to mean? The thought is fleeting and passes me by before I can tether it in my consciousness. Getting him to participate in this painful one-sided inquisition is like trying to pull teeth. *Way to throw my forty years in my face.* I am left with trying to fill in the blanks to a picture I don't even see. Now I'm angry. And I have no idea how to express this feeling that is simmering inside of me in words or in action so adept have I become at harboring resentment.

My questions feel so ridiculous in hindsight, fixated as I was on resolving a problem I had no clear image of. The pressing issue was far more a product of my then-husband's behaviors than anything that had to do with me although you might argue our dance of anger and anguish had been brewing for years. I sometimes wonder if my passion for yoga might have felt threatening to my then-husband. Or if, after my father passed away, I looked to him for something he wasn't capable of giving me, like validation or appreciation. Granted, my scorn and insults at that point did little to help my case. In the end, I found what I needed deeply imbedded within myself, excavated through years of showing up on my yoga mat working diligently to marry my mind and my body, and understanding with intuition.

Without a doubt my yoga has changed me. Not who I am, but rather, yoga has freed me up to be more myself. And this person I am now may well not have been the one my former husband thought he had married. Maybe I played small so that his light might shine brighter, but when it didn't I felt the worse for it and resentment seeped in. Maybe I played the victim to his villain, the enabler to his addictions, a defender of the very actions he took that stabbed me right in the back of my heart. Maybe it is just that my insecurities and primal fears played out their parts to perfection on the stage of our apocalyptic marriage. At the end of the day, all of this is incidental. All I needed now was to remember my own truth. Eight years after 9/11 to the day, in a muddle of confusion and anger and fear and pain, I begged out of our marriage. This was my valiant effort to reclaim myself.

This date was no accident. It was symbolic: The suffering of change and impermanence. There was the familiar tautness of my body as if to arm myself with strength and courage, accompanied by the concurrent tears of something loosening within me; and that heaviness in my heart of not wanting to let go of everything I knew. I didn't want to be charged with this decision to undo my marriage—the stakes were too high, children involved, and doing something other than everything else I had already tried meant tearing their world apart at the seams. But I dove. I dove into the unknowable and total uncertainty of 'what next?' Tears streaming, I repeated, "I can't do this anymore. I can't play this charade."

I had held onto this sinking ship of our marriage long enough. Now I had to let go. I had to make way for something else—uncertain, scary, and unknown. I had undermined myself time and time again by focusing my energies on my deficiencies (and his too, no doubt), rather than embracing everything I now have come to know and appreciate about myself including all the stuff that isn't so perfect. I forgive the past and all the moments that have passed knowing that I did my best at the time. Our imperfections, it turns out, make the perfect substrate for yoga practice.

We all have these truths that stare us down. Our yoga capitalizes on the way we feel to reveal our 'blind spots' to us, those dynamics we can't see because we are habituated to them. Through yoga, I can explore my breath when it catches in my throat, the sensation of throbbing in my chest, that feeling of ants crawling on my skin to gain a more profound understanding of how I embody stress. By the same token I learn to become more familiar and less fearful of its manifest presence in my body and to observe the ways in which my thoughts spin out into chaos so that I may, gently, corral them back to some modicum of order.

I can't mislead you now, dear yogini, and claim I was looking to live a more honest and authentic version of myself even though my soul was clamoring for it. The truth is I could no longer bear the feeling of disconnect within me that reflected itself wholeheartedly in my marital relationship under the burden of pretense and the veneer of "life is good." Here I will give my practice credit for giving me permission to feel what needed to be felt, although the clarity of "*samadhi*," the all-elusive 'True Self', had yet to reveal itself to me.

Faced with this overwhelming reality of my marriage and family falling apart at the seams I set out on the path of trying to recover who I believed myself to be. It was as if I were two separate people, this grown-up me with all the awareness of myself I have gleaned through my yoga, taking in this far younger and naïve me, dazed and confused and uncomprehending and insecure and unloved and unlovable. I could feel the bewilderment within myself and didn't know how to reconcile the knowing and empathic me with this dear, sweet, broken exiled self.

In ignorance, I continued to seek out benign assurances and validation from my former spouse, the very person who would never give it to me. During this time an angel walked into my life. Her name was Mary, a neuropsychologist by training. We connected like the two wings of a bird. Too many times I would find myself on the receiving end of that weary look of hers that read, with the utmost compassion, *You poor soul, you still don't see it do you?* Out loud in her Texan twang, "Why do you keep looking for water in the same old well honey? It's dry. If you want water, you've got to go find yourself another well, preferably one with water in it." The best advice I ever got mind you.

Practice by practice, I'd cultivate my handstand as a way to shift my perspective. Translated from the Sanskrit, handstand literally means 'upside-down-tree'. One morning I showed up on my mat, and there, lying in *supta padangustasana*, tears softly surrendered themselves, an atmospheric expression of my grief and sadness and loneliness. Yoga has this unique capacity to wear down the strata upon which our lives have been built to see ourselves more clearly. We are merely diamonds in the rough craving a good polish. As we begin to "polish" ourselves through yoga we move towards the truth of who we are, the brilliant diamond of the Self: Not the "Who?" But the "I-Am."

The Self, as a diamond, gains brilliance from three things: reflection, refraction and dispersion. Reflection is the light of consciousness that hits the 'diamond' and bounces back up, giving insight into its very nature—I call these instances "moments of *samādhi*"— instantaneous shine. This glimmer is only the very tip of the true radiance the diamond of the True Self displays. In these instances, it is easy to fall into the trap of believing, "I am enlightened." But only a portion of the light hitting our diamond is reflected; the rest travels right through it.

Refraction then is the light that moves through the diamond, scattered and fractured by tiny, complicated prisms—all the 'angles' and complexities of our being—that create the 'sparkle' that diamonds are known for. This in turn creates a dispersive rainbow effect which adds to the shine. I think of refraction and dispersion as temperament and personality, and then what we do with that is behavior. What is interesting is that, depending on where the light hits along the surface planes of the diamond, refraction and dispersion create natural areas of light and dark in the refracted light (the light that isn't reflected, or 'bounced back'). In the same vein, different stimuli affect each of us differently depending upon the angle of 'entry' engendering a positive or negative reaction with the potential to show us something that needs to be seen (reflection).

While the shadows in the shine seem counter to the brilliance we seek, really they are the magic needed to access our innate "shininess." The dark magnifies the intensity of the light; it is the candle's flame which appears brighter in the dark of night than it does in a sunlit room. Yoga boils down to contrast, to evoking the yin and the yang. Without contrast you might still shine just as bright, but then your light would be lacking the characteristic of *tapas*, the fire of transformation required so that the True Self may shine with radiance. Without this fire, we end up getting in our own way because of our resistance to what is–the proverbial mid-life crisis, or, in my case, the dissolution of a marriage in which I was blind to its inherent flaws.

Atha yogānuśāsanam. And now begins the practice of yoga.

After many years now of practice, I have become more adept at recognizing how my body reflects back to me the ease of flow and the stickiness of my resistance, and how my mind recognizes the refracted dispersion of light and the lurking shadows for what they are. Yoga is not a thinking process. It is an unfoldment of our innate somatic intelligence and the knowing of intuition, the shining of all facets of our diamond-Self so that the light of consciousness may show us more clearly to ourselves.

I see a far more discerning reflection of myself in the face of the hardships and pivotal moments that showed up in my life. As painful as it has been at times, the path through my resistance is leading me towards greater personal freedom. In the fourth book of his yoga sutras, Patañjali calls this liberation of our consciousness from the incessant and often very creative narratives of the mind, *kaivalya.* Yoga provides the tools to evaluate the assumptions we make, the expectations we impose upon ourselves, and all the other stories we tell ourselves to make sense of our own state of being, our relationships to others and the world at large. The work of yoga is not a given. You do have to show up for the practice and be willing to walk the path. Is the promise of a state of being undisturbed by life's dualities and iterations not a compelling argument to show up for oneself?

Yesterday, dear yogini, I awoke with thoughts of the past, of my regrets and chagrins, of my failure at finding happiness in the places I so desperately wanted it most, of the buried feelings that have been rising, lethargically, to the surface, to meet all those desires and dreams yet to be fulfilled...

Tomorrow I shall awake with positive imaginings for all the future holds, for a world wide open to possibility, for the potential that exists within each and every human being, for the love that buoys all of humanity…

And Today, I awake to the chirping of sunrise. I awake to the scent of Spring on the breeze of dawn. I awake to the laughter of children playing as only children can. I awake to the touch of radiance from the rising sun. I awake to the insight that everything is as it ought to be, that my questions will receive answers on the time-space continuum, and that, at this very moment, all I have to do is be present. Today I do not harbor anger or resentment. Today I do not worry—worry is but a contraption of the mind thinking about tomorrow. Today I assume personal responsibility for my life and show up with integrity for my practice. Today I shall treat all beings with kindness and respect. Today I am grateful for everyone and everything, that each may shine their unique brilliance, in shadow and in light.

Sincerely yours,

Nicole

CHAPTER 3

Dharma

"True yoga is not about the shape of your body, but the shape of your life. Yoga is not to be performed; yoga is to be lived. Yoga doesn't care about what you have been; yoga cares about the person you are becoming. Yoga is designed for a vast and profound purpose, and for it to be truly called yoga, its essence must be embodied."
– Aadil Palkhivala

February 15, 2019

Dear Yogini,

One of the most humbling aspects of yoga practice is that there is no rushing the process. As well-intentioned or driven as you may be, you actually do not get to say when, where, and how things shift and change. The more something fails to meet your expectation of it, the easier it is to get caught up in the discontent that is bound to follow, and that something then risks becoming the driver of your actions.

In this, your body becomes the ground from which you begin to explore being courageous, and every action you commit to that strengthens the resolve of the heart, your *sankalpa*. (2) Yoga becomes the way you reengage with the world to create harmony and healing. It is how you and I participate and create relationship. It does not mean you dive into a situation without forethought. On the contrary, yoga is asking you to be curious, to look at what is going on, and to train your attention to actively engage in and connect with the process.

Engagement happens on many layers, starting with the material world and at the physical level with *asana*, or posture. You maximize *asana* to enhance your sense of well-being, reduce your reactivity to stress and to work towards a balance of physical strength and mobility. As an embodied practice, *asana* is a tool like any other on the path of yoga that serves to place the attention on the inner state. The somatic feedback it offers guides and refines the yoga practice…

However, when *asana* is used as a device to achieve some external ideal or goal without suitably addressing the needs or requirements of the practitioner, call it what you will but it is bound to dilute the yogic experience. Many try yoga on for size only to conclude it is not for them for reasons of injury, overwhelm, feelings of ineptitude or insufficiency. In these instances, the *asana* experience sets illusory expectations that are not consistently realistic for the practitioner. For every person who decides that yoga is "not for me," there is a teacher who has not received the appropriate training to meet their individual need, and two more yoga practitioners like yourself debating whether to be a yoga teacher or not who will want to take this understanding into account. (12)

Perhaps it is time to shift the paradigms around misleading assumptions and negative experiences of *asana,* as much for teachers-in-training as for the yoga practitioner. Can we grow our interoceptive awareness by choosing a more conscious and refined engagement of *asana* that invites rather than imposes the somatic experience?

You and I both have an understanding that every pose unfolds at its own pace for each and every practitioner of yoga, depending upon commitment to practice, physical prowess, somatic intelligence and, of course, the *asana's* complexity. The essential poses are named after elements of nature whose qualities they embody, like *vrkshasana* (*vriksha*/tree and *asana*/pose), which integrates the solidity and steadiness of the tree rooted to the earth. Then we move into the territory of the animal kingdom where postures become somewhat more intense as they mimic or assimilate the idea of that creature's behavior or essence, like *kurmasana* (*kurma*/turtle or tortoise), a seated forward bend named for an animal that withdraws into its shell when startled or threatened and which, by design, is intended to shut out sensory distractions and quiet the nervous system; or *nakrasana* (crocodile pose) which mimics crocodilian locomotion. Finally we venture into the realm of Indian sages and avatars (rooted in Hindu mythology) whose character traits and temperaments are embodied in the postures that serve to represent them, as in *Natarajasana* (Nataraja, "the Lord of Dance") where in any one of a number of variations, Lord Shiva's dancing avatar symbolizes the cosmic cycles of birth (creation) and death (destruction) stamping out the ignorance from our minds through the divine act of dance.

Another, *Virabhradrasana* (*vira*/hero, *bhadra*/friend), the classic 'warrior pose,' is named after a mythic warrior arisen from the ground where Lord Shiva, one of the Hindu trinity of gods, supreme ruler of the universe, throws down a lock of his hair and beats it to the ground upon hearing of his wife's demise at her father's yagna, or great ritual sacrifice. There, Shiva's creation, Virabhadra, vows to destroy the powerful priest Daksha and all his guests. After Daksha fails to invite his youngest daughter, Sati, and her consort, Shiva, to his ritual offering, so the myth goes, Sati finds out and decides to go alone, then enters into an argument with her father and, unable to withstand his insults, vows: "*Since it was you who gave me this body, I no longer wish to be associated with it,*" and throws herself into the fire.

While Virabhadra first seeks to avenge the death of his wife, he later becomes understood as a symbol of dharma. When Shiva sees the chaos that his creation Virabhadra has wrought, Shiva absorbs Virabhadra back into his own form and then transforms into Hara, the ravisher. Filled with sorrow and compassion, Shiva finds Daksha's body and gives it the head of a goat, which brings him back to life. Sati too becomes reborn.

Do the various warrior stances of *Virabhadrasana*, for example, not embody your question with their invitation, in practice, to discover within yourself the courage (*vira*) to transform the personal struggles of the ego into finding purposefulness and significance in living? You know that yoga is more than a stance or a stretch or a bend in an unfathomable direction. Your practice asks more of you than mere physical prowess. It is a simple fact that *how* you live your life manifests itself in how you approach your practice. If you live your life full speed ahead, you will find yourself applying the same high-velocity temperament to your practice. It follows then that any shift in the dynamic of your life is a corollary to the conscious shifts you bring to your approach of yoga.

As your practice becomes your laboratory and your mat a test-tube of sorts, you will start to see how it is you engage with yourself in practice and thus how you comport yourself in your life. It is from this vantage point that you can stand in yourself, in yoga, to see yourself more clearly. The journey of yoga guides you through your inner states to the center of yourself. It is no accident that the struggles that show up on the mat are metaphors for the inner battles, the things we all struggle with within ourselves in the refracted light and the lurking shadows. Your practice is an opportunity for you to become the heroine of your own life. This, dear yogini, is courage.

Yoga is the process you engage in to understand your body and how it moves, to see your mind and its machinations, and to tune into the subtle and intricate complexities of how the mind and body communicate with one another. Notice how your sense perceptions and thinking can take you down the rabbit hole of distraction and distress. Whether it's music played in class or perceived shortcomings of the body or physique that undermine your exertion, your bringing your attention back (to the subtlest movement, to the coming and going of your breath, to every sensation and each moment's experiences) invites you to witness your reactivity to what is.

Pay close attention the next time music is played in your yoga class. This can be either an asset or an irritant to your practice. Sometimes the music is conducive to enhancing the experience of your practice; sometimes it dissuades you from discerning the more discriminatory effects of your exertion. You may find it offensive or triggering which sets off a reactive chain of *samsāra*, emotional and mental wanderings that preclude you from being with the somatic experience of your practice at all. It is also possible, on the other hand, that you remain oblivious to its presence throughout, although there may come a moment when the strains of melody or song permeate your consciousness. Whether music enhances your practice experience or detracts from it, start from your initial point of observation—the moment you notice any sensate reactions or feelings—to bring yourself back with ease to your breath. Placing the attention on the breath in the subtlest way allows you to create space, so you are no longer in constant service to the stimuli. The breath is quite an ingenious tool in yoga because it mimics the nature of your thoughts in its perpetual motion yet is easier to access, manipulate and manage than the mind. This is a vastly different experience from that of watching TV from the relative place of detachment you necessarily adopt with the mechanical repetition of your footfall on a Stairmaster or treadmill!

As you practice yoga, ask yourself, *How does this feel in my body? What are these thoughts? What is this story? How about this sensation or feeling that has come up? How can I work with this?* The subtle art of questioning is a way to engage your attention and direct your mind on the breath, on your thoughts, on the sensations that come up with a quality of curiosity rather than judgment.

The process begins with the attention and choosing to place it upon a specific object. In *asana*, I might place my attention on the action of my feet in a standing posture and notice how it affects the stability of my pelvis; in breath work, I might focus my attention upon the steady stream of my breath moving through me and observe its effect on my mind; in sitting practice, I might sit with my monkey mind and witness its nature. The mere act of paying attention effects demonstrable change at the most microscopic level.

This physical principle illuminates the power of the mind to affect a shift in energy dynamic when placed upon an object such as an aspect of the physiology in *asana*. In downward-facing dog pose, for instance, you can ask your abdomen to engage by drawing the naval towards the spine and this creates an energy dynamic that supports the lengthening of the lower back muscular framing the lumbar spine, nurtures the kidneys and sends a wave off energy to the realm of the heart and lungs inviting the chest cavity to feel more spacious.

In the same vein, the nerve cells, or neurons, in the human brain have the capacity to reorganize and repattern with repetition and frequency over time and form new neural connections throughout life in response to a change in their environment. This means that the repetitive nature of yoga practice has the capacity to repattern the way our muscles drive action in the physical body when we apply a discerning quality of consciousness to said action. Without this mindful application of our awareness to the ways in which we engage our physical actions, the rote performance of *asana* in yoga practice risks reinforcing the very patterns of stress in our lives that we carry in our bodies and that then show up in our practice.

Thus, yoga is a process of direct experimentation used to explore your observations and answer your questions, much like the scientific method. Yoga is science based on Samkhya philosophy, which is the very basis of all sciences. (3) Samkhya translates as "that which explains the whole" and embraces the whole universe—how the universe came into existence and all relationships within the universe. It explains human life on all levels which is why yoga is such a potent path to resolving your dilemma.

Where yoga holds particular vigor is in the knowledge gleaned through the sensate experiences of posture, the breath, the mind, the intellect, and overall awareness that understands something to be true because it has been directly perceived. It may not always make sense to your faculties of reason. And so, by heightening your powers of direct perception, you test and cultivate your ability to feel your muscles and bone, to tune into the subtleties of your breath, to witness your mental fluctuations, then to directly perceive the still subtler energy shifts of your inner being and eventually that deepest seat of the Self, the quality of spirit or that something intangible yet comforting and sweet.

This paradigm is affirmed by Patañjali in the first chapter of *The Yoga Sūtras* (YS I.7) which essentially informs us that "correct knowledge" is based on three types of evidence: direct perception (through direct experience), reasoning (through inference or deduction) and trusted testimony from a higher authority. I can personally attest to the power of direct perception: Everything I teach I know to be true because of my direct experience with it. It is a spectacular process once you learn to trust it. There is a powerful word in the Sanskrit language that expresses this epistemology: *Śraddhā,* a faith born from experience, or more literally, as anything or any act that is performed with all sincerity. To engage *śraddhā,* you must learn to trust yourself.

Yoga, as a science, a philosophy, and a practice, asks you to partake with consistency and dedication in a process of observation to connect with the unchangeable Self which sees reality as it is. From this vantage point of seeing clearly what is, you can stand in trust of yourself and participate in conscious relationship with the world. You learn how to be at peace with difficulty and how to embrace joy. You become skillful at managing expectations and engage with your life as a friend rather than an enemy. You also understand that yoga changes your relationship with yourself. As a result, you may lose friends or loved ones who, out of their own discomfort or intolerance, cannot or will not abide these changes.

The Yogic Wisdom is the path to solving your dilemma, my friend, as you learn to trust in yourself along the way. Forgive me, dear yogini, if you already have a fundamental understanding of Patañjali's classical eight-faceted path of Yoga (delineated in *sutras II.28-34*) as the path the yogin takes to shift the arc of their life towards freedom and peace.

Given all the emphasis placed on physical practice in the West, note that Patañjali falls somewhat short on describing *asana*, or 'posture' in his yoga sutras. Of course, there are plenty of other texts that reference a system of physical techniques (notably Svāmi Svātmārāma's Hatha Yoga Pradipikā, which outlines yoga in four stages or chapters). There is, too, a wonderful collection of verses of the Indian sage Gheranda (known as the Gheranda Samhita) that sets itself apart from other texts on hatha yoga with its reference to the 'person' rather than the 'body.' In this, Sage Gheranda teaches his disciple, King Chandakapali, techniques that work on the body and the mind in the context of a seven-fold path to the realization of the Self. Like other root hatha yoga texts, however, the Gherana Samhita does not appear to concern itself much with the ten precepts that make up the first two facets of Patañjali's classical Yoga.

The continuous exploration and exploitation of Patañjali's fundamental precepts—*yama*, or moral restraint, rooted in the reflection of our true nature, and *niyama*, or personal observances, (4) rooted in our evolution towards harmony—invite the practical application of Yogic Wisdom to unfold in the context of life itself. *Yama* and *niyama* serve to polish the multi-faceted surfaces of yoga practice and experience, as a diamond is cut to produce the ultimate brilliance and fire. In applying these precepts to your yoga, with specific attention to your thoughts and your ways of seeing, you will change the relationship you have with yourself. You will alter the relationship you have with others, and you will recast the relationship you have with the world as you come to terms with how you resolve your question.

The third facet, or *asana*, the physical aspect of your practice must include equal measures of persistent effort to realize the objective of self-knowing and a corresponding release of attachment to the stuff that stands in the way. This might manifest as striving for standards of external accomplishment, listening to the 'shoulds' and the 'cannots' decided by your ever-fickle mind, or quashing the traumas and tragedies of the heart that have taken up residence in your body and are stored in your subconscious. All of it bubbles up at the end of the day, if not on your yoga mat, then in your life. So perhaps it is not such a bad thing if you can take the seat of *asana* and act upon your body with wisdom. Notice the distractions, the discouragements and the boredom that are an inevitable component of practice, and allow those unprocessed stories and emotions behind them to rise up and occasionally disturb the smooth layer of platitudes that protect your inner realm.

Add to this some modulation of the breath, or *prāṇāyāma*, the fourth facet of Yogic Wisdom. You breathe, you pay attention to your breath, and you vary your breathing patterns with *pranayama*, techniques to remember to be intensely present to what you are doing and what you feel in the moment. Our consciousness is colored by our attachments to sense objects such as our environment, people, ideas, opinions, narratives, and other such things. The breath serves to control the senses by drawing them inwards to focus on the more subtle movements of prana under the surface layer of awareness. *What does it mean to control the senses, and what import does this have in yoga practice?*

This is *pratyahara*, the fifth facet of the path you are on. When you have little control over how you respond or react to external stimuli you are at the behest of your conditioned tendencies or habits, referred to in yoga as *samskaras*, you risk defining yourself by the nature of your experience, thereby taking things personally. This means you will avoid pain and gravitate towards all things pleasurable, unable to hold the space between stimulus and response. Unlike the intellect, which operates along the lines of reasoning, your understanding moves from looking out to seeing in, from outer listening to inner hearing—tuning into that quiet voice that will serve you in your quest for an answer to a specific question—to kinesthetic sensitivity in the deepest layers of your being, to savoring the air you breathe.

This, in turn, develops the sixth facet, concentration or contemplation. This is called *dhāranā*. In the first sutra of book III of the *Yoga Sūtras*, Patañjali states that gathering consciousness and focusing it within is *dharana*, or contemplation; you are beginning to transition from the realm of practice, per se, to progressive internal states that evolve from the earlier cultivated practices, facets of the yogic path that have been 'shined' by your consciousness. The same attention and awareness that is present in *dharana* is also brought to *dhyana*, meditation, the seventh facet of the yogic path, as to the initial states of *samadhi*, the eighth facet, seeing clearly things as they are. Eventually perhaps, total absorption is achieved—the ability to rest in the spirit of *purusha*, to step into the power of perceiving reality as it is, where the coverings, deceptions, illusions, and contraptions of the mind fall away and the light of consciousness shines through.

Analogous to the clarity of a diamond, which refers to the absence of inclusions and blemishes, so does the Self shine when we bleach our consciousness of its colorings. This is not to say that you have to abandon your possessions, your friends or beliefs. Yoga simply asks that you recognize their transitory character and release yourself of those that no longer serve you when the appropriate time comes to do so. This is something I needed to do for myself by releasing myself of the bonds of a marriage that denigrated vows I took to heart. Patañjali states, in *sutra I.41*, that our consciousness becomes like a "polished crystal" (5) that allows the light of our authentic Self, the *atman*, to shine through brilliantly without distortion.

I make frequent reference to Patañjali as the forefather of yoga as we know it here in the West so as to neither dilute the teachings of yoga or to misappropriate the richness of all that yoga offers. My wish is to make these age-old wisdom teachings and powerful practices accessible and applicable to contemporary life for it is here you will find resolution to your question. I share with you my experiences and understanding of the science and art and methodology that is yoga to show you that yoga works. Your yoga will inform your life, and your life will inform your yoga. It works both ways. I hold the candid belief that no matter how life shows up for you your sincere embodiment of the essence of yoga will serve you in living into an answer to your question.

Eventually, dearest yogini, your resolute and vigilant enterprise on the yoga mat will lead you to a clear resolution of your dilemma for the simple reason you will become clear on your thoughts rather than identify with them in mistaken or confused understanding.

Peace and beautiful practice.

Sincerely yours,

Nicole

CHAPTER 4

The Discipline of Yoga

"Yoga is a light, which once lit, will never dim.
The better your practice, the brighter the flame."
– B.K.S. Iyengar

Winchester, MA—February 25, 2019

Dear Yogini,

As I give considerations to the context in which I use the term yoga, I find myself curious to know your take on this too. When talking about yoga, would you say something like "I do yoga," "I study yoga," or "I practice yoga?" This might help you clarify your intention behind the question, "Is teaching yoga for me or not?" There are, of course, many distinctions to be made with respect to the term yoga, but the point I am making is that it would be so easy to fall into a clichéd use of the word "yoga" and any and all the physical, spiritual, or other stereotypes and assumptions—true and false—associated with its common usage. So I ought not to assume but rather request clarification from you of what you understand yoga to be.

I keep returning to Patañjali's opening aphorism, *Atha yogānuśāsanam*: Here and now begins the discipline of yoga, "the containment of one's ways of thought." Inherent in the methodology of the eight-limbed path of yoga described by Patañjali is the disciplinary aspect. Yoga is an engagement, a contract of sorts with your Self, a powerful way to change how a situation unfolds by the way you perceive it (and bring consciousness to it) or by the way you think about it (and bring intentionality to that thinking).

Instead of seeing life as simply happening to you, you have the option of being an active participant in the process of life, and yoga becomes an invitation to get off the sidelines, to stop being passive—a doormat or victim of circumstance or just plain playing small—and take action. Your participation creates the possibility of a different outcome, a shift in dynamics, transmuting weakness into strength, self-preoccupation into self-awareness, self-absorption into compassion. Your involvement affects how the "game" unfolds; you influence the outcome by your mere presence and intentionality of heart.

Do you recall the precepts I alluded to in my previous letter? While every religion, every dogma has their own version of such guidelines for moral behavior, I believe these to be neither doctrine nor dogma. My training is in the biological sciences so I take nothing at face-value, including the instruction and origins of the practice of yoga.

Vyasa, the original interpreter of *The Yoga Sūtras*, divided Patanjali's compilation of Yogic Wisdom into four books, which some argue is "artificial and incorrect. (6)" I have alternated between contemplating Indian philosophy and applying its precepts to my life throughout the last two decades of my personal and professional engagement with this discipline of yoga. It is in this context I hope to frame for you, and for myself too, this profound and potent Yogic Wisdom.

And so we have a path that came to be known as *asta-anga* ("eight-limbed") *yoga* (referenced in *sutra II.29*). The Sanskrit word for ashtanga (transliterated with the additional 'h' for pronunciation's sake), is derived from the words 'astha,' "eight" and 'anga,' typically translated as "limb" or "facet." While this 'eight-limbed' path of yoga gives the impression of linearity, it is in fact, evidenced by my own experience of the practice, an integrated system of tenets (*yama*, the five abstentions or restraints, with a focus towards minding our behavior in the world, and *niyama*, the five observances, with a focus towards caring for ourselves), physical activity, breath, sensory awareness and withdrawal, concentration, mind observation, and absorption. James Haughton Woods in his annotation of the sutras refers to these as the "eight aids of yoga (7)"—the first five facets as "indirect aids" to yoga (*yama, niyama, āsana, prānāyāma* and *pratyahara*) which, in my understanding, are loosely referenced as "hatha yoga" because they extend ways to balance the solar and lunar dynamics inherent in all our physiological and energetic systems; and the latter three facets—to do with mind control—as "direct aids" to yoga (*dhāranā, dhyana* and *samādhi*) which, together, are alluded to as "raja yoga," the 'royal' path.

Thus, yoga is the practice of journeying inwards towards seeing and knowing Self more clearly without the camouflage of our unconscious conditioning, our arrogance and privilege, our perceived deficits, the veil of our ignorance, or our implicit socio-economic, cultural, and religious biases. Recall that the primordial instruction in the discipline of yoga is "the containment of one's ways of thought. (8)" And as the "aids" of yoga are engaged, and when the "impurities" of the mind have dwindled, there arises "an enlightenment of perception reaching up to the discriminative discernment, (9)" as stated in *sutra I.28* which describes the goal of the eight-limbed path of yoga.

So with regard to *yama* and *niyama*, the tenets of yoga—the first and second "indirect aids" to purify the mind and pave the way for enlightened perception—you get to fashion and re-fashion them according to what unfolds for you along your path; you get to revisit them at your leisure and as you see fit to do so, for there is no one single way to work with them. It is how you choose to live into these tenets that will clarify how your dilemma matures and finds resolution. *Yama* and *niyama* are the foundation of your yoga, and because yoga is not a linear process, you will tease them and defy them, work with them and refine them until you have scratched the last of the veneer off and can live these precepts as your ultimate truth.

Your personal exploration of the five inner precepts called *yama* will encourage you to live more at ease with yourself and then with others and then, God-willing, with the world at large:

- Practice being reverent and kind, practice non-violence (*ahimsa*).
- Dedicate yourself to the truth so that your thought, words, and deeds may manifest the power of this truth (*satya*).
- Give of yourself but do not compare or steal away what does not belong to you (*asteya*).
- Devote yourself to leading a balanced and sensate life in the present moment so that you live into harmony with your consciousness (*brahmacharya*).
- Count your blessings and acknowledge the abundance in your life; do not want for more than is necessary (*aparigraha*).

Your personal foray into the five precepts called *niyama* allows you to continue your journey inward toward wholeness and discovering your destiny:

- Cultivate purity, knowing your Self through simplicity and discernment so that your body, your thoughts, your emotions become clear reflections of you (*saucha*).
- Cultivate contentment by taking pause and noticing the spaces 'in-between' (*santosa*).
- Cultivate discipline with wisdom: Show up to do the work with sincerity and passion (*tapas*).
- Study, contemplate, retreat so that you may be guided to the seat of the Self (*svadhyaya*).
- And move towards the Sacred Self as a way to align yourself with your life, your dharma, and the light of universal consciousness (*Isvara pranidhana*).

These tenets are vast and continuous practices that serve but a small purpose until your heart is ready to receive them. You will need the rigors of practice to see and dissolve whatever rules and regulations you adhere to that no longer serve you, and to reframe whatever principles and paradigms have directed you in unsuitable ways. And then, dearest yogini, any confusion, any doubt, any uncertainty that enshrouds your question and whatever else is getting in your way will fade. I have no doubt your answer will be revealed to you, as you perceive reality as it is and when the opportune moment arises.

The objective of Patañjali's yoga, as detailed in his yoga sutras, is for us to recognize and realize the true nature of (Absolute) Reality—that which is not subject to change, death, and decay—and to touch the unchangeable witness within, lyricism incarnate in Rainer Maria Rilke's *Book of Hours: Love Poems to God*. Just as you can see yourself in the mirror, dear yogini, so also, through yoga *darshana* (the yoga sutras, or any 'system' through which you see reality as it is), can you see the Self. This brilliant diamond of the Self is defined here as 'pure consciousness' (or *purusha*) and is distinct from mere matter (*prakrti*) which includes the body, mind, thoughts, intellect, and temporal ego, all of which are subject to change and entirely impermanent.

I have found myself subject to the common understanding that yoga signifies "yoke" or "union." In its classical usage, the Sanskrit word for 'yoke' is *yuj* and refers to a wooden crosspiece that is fastened over the necks of two animals (in the Indian tradition, horses destined for battle), and attached to the plow or cart that they are to pull. So 'yoga,' as a device, serves to control the frenzied nervousness of war horses, the "chomping at the bit;" as a technique, yoga serves to bring two elements together, two halves of a whole: the right hemisphere of the brain with the left; the brain with the body; the sympathetic nervous system with the parasympathetic nervous system; the yin with the yang; the female and the male; the individual consciousness (or *atman*) with the universal principle (or *brahman*).

In essence, dear yogini, according to Patañjali, rather than union or oneness with the world, you seek instead to liberate yourself from your attachments to the temperamental changeability of the world's materialistic nature to become one with yourself. You and I change our minds on a whim; our thoughts come and go as they please, audacious and unbidden and too often impertinent, graceless, and of little service to our general wellbeing. Feelings arise like weather-systems, entirely out of our immediate control, supplanted by emotional interpolations that ride in on anything from the gentlest tide to the most daunting tsunami. And then, too often, we take these thoughts or emotions at face value. We begin to believe the stories we or others' tell about ourselves; God forbid we take others' perceptions and opinions and judgments of us to heart.

Instead, use the precepts, these tenets of yoga to guide you along the path of ashtanga yoga towards a clearer understanding of the question you have for yourself. May your practice of yoga serve to bring you back to the heart of You and who you wish to be in the world. Do not take others' judgments and opinions of you personally—especially when you begin to teach your yoga; you will come to learn that this is the practice of *asteya*, to not indulge the tendencies of one's ego-self or another's to create division or hierarchy of less and greater than. May you find yourself inspired by some great purpose where you are free from fear and thus the ego, where your thoughts transcend their limitations, your consciousness expands in all directions. May you, through your yoga, live your quest into its resolution.

Peace and beautiful practice.

Sincerely yours,

Nicole

"The journey of a thousand miles begins with a single step."
— **Lao-Tzu**

CHAPTER 5

Probing Conditioned Consciousness:
How Do You Want to Act in the World?

*"If you are willing to change your thinking, you can
change your feelings. If you change your feelings, you
can change your actions. And changing your actions—
based on good thinking—can change your life."*
– John C. Maxwell

Winchester, MA—February 28, 2019
Dear Yogini,

I find myself excited for you to travel this path of yoga so that your intuitive wisdom may dawn as clarity and confidence in the direction of your dreams. You strike me as a curious person by nature and that is, in my most humble opinion, the most lucrative place to start. Curiosity replaces any propensity for judgment and criticism, defensiveness and condemnation, stonewalling and denial—a waste of perfectly good energy that can be better spent moving you in the direction of your own self-mastery.

Patañjali's eight-faceted ashtanga yoga begins with exploring the reflection of the True Self (10) through *yama*. Like all facets or angles of this yogic path, each *yama* serves to 'restrain' some aspect of our conditioned behaviors and implicit biases. Each yama inhabits the same consciousness as the others, so do not consider separating one *yama* from another, dear yogini. Each one acts as a mechanism for change and is but one fragment of the whole that you seek. Can you discipline your psyche to change from hostility to humility through force of will? Have you tried to love unconditionally someone you resent? Or attempted to forgive outright someone who has done you harm? Transform envy into admiration? Then you can conceive that each facet of your practice requires consistent and continual 'shining' so that the brilliance of humility and love and forgiveness and admiration may reflect themselves in your sphere of consciousness without the weight of refracted truth undermining what they mean to you.

Ahimsa: Practice kindness and respect, practice non-harm.

Ahimsa is the opposite of violence. Generally-speaking, *ahimsa* asks us to practice kindness and respect towards all beings everywhere. *Ahimsa* is movement away from our habitual attempts to impress our will or beliefs or power onto others. Criticism, judgment, condemnation, negativity are all subtle (and sometimes not so subtle) ways in which we harm ourselves and those around us. This quality of self-talk (directed towards self and others) undermines the esteem we have for ourselves and robs us of the light that consciousness brings to our shadows. It takes bravery to face the internal strife that reflects this war inside ourselves against our very own nature. The practice of *ahimsa* asks that you take this seat of the witness and, in practice, learn to access, then rest into your tension, your pain, your hurt, your satisfactoriness, your suffering, or *dukkha*.

There was a time where I labeled my former spouse a narcissist, a cheater, and a bully to frame my experiences of emotional gaslighting and betrayal, and conversely to make sense of my own feeling of low self-worth in this relationship. While there is usually some nugget of truth in how we each frame our respective realities, labels provide a convenient, yet simplistic and limiting viewpoint to make sense of how we feel. Labels validate our emotional and/or mental states, and may help to create understanding around our experiences. Rarely do they diminish our attachment to the deleterious and sometimes destructive feelings these experiences engender within us.

Your yoga gives you permission to feel the hurt caused by the labels imposed upon you, and conversely the labels you have imposed upon yourself and others. Your consistent practice has the capacity to reflect back to you the ways in which you frame your experiences and perceived truths, and the ways too in which you habitually react. This line from the Ashtanga opening incantation, *Samsara halahala mohashantyai,* asks our practice to help us first see, then remove the poison of conditioned existence (that causes harm to ourselves and others)—these repetitive behaviors that neither inspire us nor elevate us to a greater purpose—then replace them with coherent consciousness.

We do not need to condone patterns of speech and behaviors that are hurtful, intentionally or not. We can, however, with this practice of *ahimsa*, learn to forgive so we do not marinate in resentment or anger or any of the shadow aspects of violence. If there is anything my own temporary wrath showed me, it is that this heated and contracted way of framing my reality also made me view the world outside of me-myself-and-I from a more hostile perspective. It served only to imprison me behind walls of my own making and made me more furious and less free. My level of stress skyrocketed, dysplasia imminent (in my mind), and catabolic surges of cortisol and adrenaline flooded my bloodstream triggering a state of anxiety that consumed me. This, I came to recognize, is not self-love.

Ahimsa asks us to re-evaluate these paradigms we have around any viewpoint that does not serve our best interests in a positive way. In our culture, we have societal paradigms around physical appearance and health that run deep through the fiber of our being human. So notice your process in *asana*, the physical approach to your practice. Notice how you accept your physical skill or reject your lack thereof in your postures; how you rally your good efforts and denigrate your perceived failures. The application of *ahimsa* to your physical practice calls your awareness to the heartfelt intention with which you choose to be in your body in *asana* at any given instant.

Patañjali describes the effects of observing *ahimsa* in speech, thought and action (in *sutra II.35*) as relinquishing your aggressive tendencies and inviting those in your presence to do the same. Let us all persevere in our practice of *ahimsa* to cultivate the positive qualities of the mind and attitudes of friendliness, compassion, delight, and disregard that allow the mind to remain unperturbed (*sutra I.33*).

Satya: Dedicate yourself to the truth so that your thought, words, and deeds may manifest the power of this truth.

Inherent in the understanding of *satya* (truthfulness) is the assumption that neither you nor I distort or alter in any way a truth to suit our own needs or meet the expectation of another. Not all of us, however, are clear all the time on the distinction between what our truth is and what truth belongs to another. Where there is a status differential there is always the risk of one person subjugating themselves to the truth of the authority, and conversely the authority figure imposing their truth upon their subject. It is all too common an occurrence where students (of yoga and otherwise) project their desires as well as their ineptitudes upon their teacher seeking to get their needs met by that person; conversely, not all teachers (of yoga and otherwise) are sincere in establishing firm professional boundaries as a way of creating safe space for their students. This differential creates internal dissonance.

I have certainly experienced this feeling of internal dissonance, which feels to me much as guilt and confusion do. This fundamental discord arises from the differential between the truth I think I or someone else desires (a contraption of the mind) and my shiny-diamond self-truth (the sincerity of heart), and not always knowing exactly what that is. The embodied practices of yoga are critical to putting us in touch with our deepest understanding of Self.

In conflict, we understand there to be at least two distinct, and frequently discordant, accounts of what has transpired. We are all guilty on the one hand, of internalizing the conflict as repressive tendencies (where the emotional energy behind the conflicting elements gets shut down by the mind and stored in the body as resentment and dis-ease); and on the other, of externalizing our conflict as expressive tendencies (where the emotional energy behind the conflicting elements gets directed outwardly at someone or something as blame, shame, bullying, aggression, etc.).

Yoga asks us to observe these feelings of conflict and disconnect in the moment, as they arise. This is an exacting practice. It requires a sincere dedication to challenging the status quo; a commitment to asking more *of* yourself and wanting more *for* yourself. To be with discomfort and pain is hard. Yet, the more you practice paying attention, the more familiarity you gain with the sensations and feelings behind the emotions and the energy of conflict. Every sensation that shows up, every feeling that is felt, every emotion that manifests is first filtered through the background of your own conditioning. Thought patterns and habitual reactive tendencies are entrenched in every single cell and fiber of your own being. Behind this conditioning, and colored by it, lies the truth of who you are, the diamond-brilliance. *Satya* is a practice of learning to perceive the discolorations and refractions that distort your truth, so that you may live into it.

Any attack on me or my truth and I can feel it at the level of my bones to the surface of my skin. It has an antagonistic quality to it and sets off my defense mechanisms in the form of self-righteous indignation. It turns out this is not a very attractive trait when I observe it in someone else's field of reactivity! So I notice this tendency first within myself. I pause. I breathe. I invite my sphere of awareness to illuminate these feelings, these energies, without making them anything other than what they are, nothing more than shadows lurking. The shadows still lurk, I still react, but I now have some capacity to see this, step out of my reactivity and regain perspective. This, to me, is what the practice of standing in truth looks like.

I have always been completely captivated and entirely envious of those people you come across in life who exude confidence and sincerity of being. The one thing perhaps that has worked in favor of my moving in that direction is the simple fact that I have always wanted to *be* that person. Whether you choose to become a yoga teacher or not, your perseverance in practice comes with a responsibility to embody the precepts of yoga and present yourself to your fellow practitioners, to your students, and in all your relationships in a way that is congruent with the truth of who you are. In other words, you have to keep up your own practice.

This practice works. Other than having to meet my own expectations of myself, I know now to differentiate for myself and for others, in truth, what acceptable (behavior) is and what it is not, so as not to mislead or, conversely, take another's misinterpretation of my actions to heart. I also know that failure is just another interpretation for feedback: No longer am I 'not enough' or insufficient; neither do I need to be first, or the best, or the most viable, or at the center of attention. And I certainly do not need to meet another's criterion (especially my own) of perfection. Excellent, yes; perfect, no. I can set my expectations to the level of reasonable and realistic and stand in a place of owning my own truth—regardless of anyone else's opinion of what I should do or who I should be. I want to say that again: *regardless of anyone else's opinion of what I 'should' do or who I 'should' be.*

Asteya: Do not rob yourself of that which you are deserving of, or take from another that which has not been earned.

Your biggest and most fragile liability is your ego, which seeks permanence, continuity, and certainty—none of which are real. Classical yoga calls this trait 'I-am-ness', or *asmita*, the ignorance that comes from identification with the ego. The contraption of the ego is self-limiting when we stylize or curate ourselves to meet an ideal perpetuated by our culture or another person that is incongruent with who we are. We limit ourselves when we pretend to be someone we are not; we limit ourselves by not being exactly who we are and were always meant to be—in accordance with *yama* and *niyama*, *ahimsa* and *satya*.

With the practice of *asteya*, you measure yourself against another and begin to see how you create a sophisticated dynamic of 'lesser than' and 'greater than'. You might classify your workplace as toxic, divide your family into dysfunctional or supportive, and judge your fellow yogin as adept or inept against whom you decide to measure your own self-worth. How simple it is for envy and jealousy to usurp the sense of completeness and self-sufficiency you seek to cultivate through your practice: *I want what that person has*; and not only do you not have enough, *I want that 'other' thing over there, that body, that house, that job, that life.* This means that the present moment has evaporated, and you find yourself sucked into a vortex of unexcavated envy that sours into resentment, indignation, silent condemnation, and anger. And guess what? Most of the time, the other person has no clue about how you feel.

It takes inordinate self-mastery to go into yourself to perceive the experience that emerges in the moment from your individual belief system, from your fears, from your ignorance and lack of understanding, from your desires, your temptations, your assumptions and expectations, from your past experiences and future imaginings. We define ourselves as good at yoga or not good at yoga; flexible enough or too tight to do yoga, and in this way cleave life into the duality of "me" and "the rest of the world." Our collective mistruths and grievances, subtle or overt, steal the harmony from our relationships.

I craved fulfillment in my marriage that made me seek from my spouse validation and acceptance he couldn't give me. When my insecurities bumped into his tendencies towards isolation and self-denial, I believed myself to be unattractive, unloved, and completely insignificant. How I lacked the understanding to see myself separate from all those vacuous markers of self-worth! It makes me so sad to think this is how I once perceived myself and that my standards for self-worth and self-love reached so low.

In essence, I had to learn to befriend myself again, to probe beneath my lack of fulfillment and find its cause. I had to look long and hard at this tendency to steal from myself and give to another, to play small so that someone else's light might shine brighter. And understand why I felt the imperative to acquire knowledge and expertise so that I might feel sufficient, enlightened perhaps and quite possibly superior. And I had to finally acknowledge the position of privilege I was born into just by being White and didn't realize I occupied until I was called out by a gentle and compassionate friend; I still have to work at this practice of standing in that 'other' person's shoes to see the world from their point of view and experience, more so Today than ever before.

Everyone falls into the habit of dividing and classifying the world into comparative parts because we think that the accumulation of wealth, the acquisition of knowledge or certification, losing weight, being a more accomplished yogi will always appear to provide fulfillment where it lacks. Pride and lust and greed build complex walls of made-up stories and ideals, securities and safety systems, pontifical abuse of power and privilege, diagnostics, and diagnoses behind which we hide from our unwillingness to see and acknowledge the truth when it is revealed to us. When you stand up and say out loud, *I am not going to participate in this anymore,* this is *asteya*, literally 'non-stealing.'

Brahmacharya: Devote yourself to leading a balanced and sensate life, in the present moment, so that you live into harmony with your consciousness.

We experience life through our senses, do we not? Close your eyes for a moment. What sensate memory awakens in you a quality of desire, pleasure, or transportation? Is it the sweet carriage of rose in summer? The succulent taste of honey or the bitter, full-flavor of coffee on your tongue? The soothing sounds of the ocean impressed upon your consciousness? An image of color and beauty cast in film upon your retina and imprinted in the recesses of your visual cortex? The felt sense of touch, of silk or velvet or other soft pleasure against your skin? Do you see how beauty and joy and sensuality occur when we are in the moment? We abandon all these possibilities of spontaneous élan when we are instead seeking excitation of the senses, mere transitory pleasure, immediate gratification.

In the classic wisdom of yoga, this practice is referred to as *brahmacharya*, a concept within Indian religions that literally means "conduct consistent with Brahma." In simple terms, *brahmacharya* is the path of Brahma, or universal consciousness, where the yogini controls her *città* (mental fluctuations or processes) in order to moderate her words, thoughts, and actions with respect to the gravitational draw of physical, sensate, and sensual pleasures. More commonly translated as "celibacy," one can hardly expect today's yogin to refrain altogether from sexual activity.

However, I raise the point because confusion and misunderstanding, personal struggles, and abuse of discretion abound where sexual issues are concerned, not just in the general realm but in yoga too. How many so-called gurus have exploited their positions of power, their gift of privilege, and their points of access in pursuit of gratification of the senses and sexual proclivities? *What does being a teacher of yoga mean, to you?*

This question is significant not just in terms of how it relates to sexuality and gratification and attachment to the limiting values of the ego but in how teachers of yoga, now more than ever, must uphold the tenets of yoga as an example to their students. Patañjali's code of ethics exposes all of the human condition and shows us that we are all fallible as human beings. Have you looked at what gratification and sex and desire means in your life? How has it shown up in the past? Is it relevant? Are we, as a culture, doing the work of peeling back the layers and observing ourselves in action? Can we perceive that which lies at the root of our distortions and delusions of desire? What is it within us that is seeking to be discovered, uncovered, and recovered?

Think about this for a moment, dear yogini. That you are seeking to know more about your yoga and the Yogic Wisdom says to me that you are already in a process of self-reflection and perhaps willing too to shift something primordial within yourself to access your truth. This is how you come to find yourself in the midst of your dilemma working from a vast collection of memories and karmic experiences in reach of some desired outcome, acting now upon that desire. This is how you find yourself in the middle of a question that can only be lived into in the present; otherwise, the present becomes a way to fashion the future according to some ideal or power play in your head or replay of some past experience. In essence, all your difficulties are created by this division of your experiences into time.

There are never enough hours in the day, dear yogini, not enough weeks in the calendar year, no empty space in daily life in which to 'not-think' or 'do', and so little time to do everything that needs to be done. All of this precludes us living right here into this breath, into this moment, and then when the time comes, into the next. If you cannot resolve your dilemma, dearest yogini, how can anyone else possibly resolve it for you? Self-discovery, yogic wisdom teaches, can only occur in relationship to the present moment. At every moment, you are capable of looking at yourself, your thoughts, your feelings, and the way you act and behave. You have a teacher, you seek a teacher, or you want to be a teacher. No matter. Remember simply that you are your own best teacher for leading and inspiring your journey along this path, for yoga invites you to know yourself better than anyone else possibly can or ever will.

Aparigrapha: Count your blessings and practice living life to its fullest.

The principles of behavior that Patañjali places before us enable us to be 'in' the world rather than 'of' the world. *Aparigraha* is the fifth *yama* and offers us an opportunity to practice not getting too attached to the idea of 'more.' The ego and its grasping and clinging and wanting for something 'other than' creates walls that imprison us within the confines of our, by nature, self-limiting perspectives. Have you never craved a little 'more' from your yoga practice—more ease, more flexibility, more power, more stature, to be 'more' like someone else—and then tried to squeeze yourself into some uncomfortable ideal or concept (of a pose or the practice itself) that doesn't meet your needs or feel good?

Yoga tells us that this entrapment in the illusions of needing 'more'— and we can always use more confidence, more money, more fame, more attention or validation or love, etc.—is nothing but a fearful operation that craves permanence, a sense of safety and security. The problem then becomes our dependence on outside forces for our satisfaction and sense of fulfillment. We can want for all of the things in the world but add to that our attachment to an ideal or concept we've been sold, and we risk striving for something that isn't real and then suffering the distress of losing something we never had in the first place.

Consider all the things that we reach for outside ourselves that illustrate this precept only too well: Food, alcohol, drugs, sex, fame, fortune, social media, material goods, our looks, are all such examples. Your yoga asks you to refine the positive qualities of the mind that breed respect and friendliness (*ahimsa*), to stand in your own brilliance (*satya*) and align yourself with your indivisible truth (*asteya*), and practice conduct consistent with who you are in truth (*brahmacharya*) so that you can stand solid in the midst of temptations and ideals that distort or draw you away from who you know yourself to be (*aparigraha*).

We can take action and hold onto the promise of a specific outcome with the risk of defaulting to our original state a little worse for wear. And we can elevate ourselves to gain recognition risking a bruised ego. Until we explore the root causes of our attachments and come to see them for what they are—greed, vanity, success, affirmation, security, etc.—any attempt to create non-attachment only strengthens the source of our attachment.

So in your practice of yoga, dear yogini, persevere at assuming ownership for the choices you make. It is not the choice itself that is subject to scrutiny in practice but rather the attitude with which you approach the choice you make and the sincerity behind it. Ask yourself this in practice: Is your decision intentional? Is your choice colored by craving? Do you seek individuality (not inherently a bad thing)? And if so, is there a something underneath that individuality that seeks to perpetuate continuity, immortality, or that fragment of thought that divides the world into me and not-me, mine and not-mine? Are you cultivating a relationship with the world around you that preserves your independence? Are you stepping into the world without possessiveness?

I experience *aparigraha* as a practice of simplification, of reducing my needs to only the most essential elements. I can't say it is an easy practice, but I have learned that when I don't hold on so tight to everything I cherish, and learn to loosen my grip on it, then I get to experience firsthand the full impact of my attachment. With each and every takeaway I have learned a little more about myself.

My largest lesson in this practice of *aparigraha* has been to value my self-worth and to not compromise myself. Nothing in this material world of ours can define your self-worth. You will want to take all that yoga is teaching you on the mat into living *your* life, and not let the world (or anyone in it) define you and who you believe yourself to be. You are not defined by your body; you are not defined by your posture; you are not defined by how hard or well or far you travel in your practice. You are only defined by how well you have learned to love and to live your life, informed by the lessons gleaned in learning to 'let go'. This realization is *aparigraha*.

Like *atman* (your true self), the sun shines its continuous light. Anything that covers your innate brilliance or anyone who turns you away from the sun denies you the ability to see your true nature. When your thoughts and emotions cloud the mind, you only suffer for not seeing the sun. Perceive the contents of your mind for what they are, and notice too the ways in which your thoughts seek some semblance of constancy and sameness, holding onto outdated paradigms and tales that do not belong to you. Your practice becomes one of carefully teasing apart the fragile construction of your habitual thinking and daily existence. Practice the abundance of *aparigraha* to replace what must be let go of.

As you travel the path of yogic wisdom you will refine what it is you are seeking for yourself in yoga, and as you do so, you will start living into the answers to all your questions including the ones you have yet to ask. You need not know your direction or destination, but without a firm understanding of yourself and how you want to be in the world, how are you to resolve your dilemma? How are you to relate to others? How are you to explore the ever-widening aspects and divisions of our outer world?

The practice of *ahimsa* only dissolves the violence of our culture and our self-hatred once we have perceived what lies at the root of it, within ourselves. The practice of *satya* only disperses the lies, deceit, and dishonesty when that which lies at their root has been perceived. *Asteya* emerges from the dissolution of our sophisticated paradigms of comparison that divide and isolate each of us from the other. The practice of *brachmacharya* tames the pangs of pleasure and immediate gratification until self-realization is arrived at by degrees. And *aparigraha* teaches us to let go little by little of the things that get in the way of our perceiving our inner truth and the light of our collective consciousness. These are the principles of *yama*.

Niyama then takes us on an inbound journey to the center of our personal solar system where *atman*, or soul, abides. The practice of *niyama* now serves to purify our physical, energetic, mental, and intellectual sheaths, or *koshas*, of the debris that obscures the light of spirit. Then perhaps we can perceive Self as connected to the vaster realm of consciousness, that 'something' larger than ourselves that Patañjali refers to in the yoga sutras as *Ishvara*. Let this be the topic of our next encounter, dear yogini. Until then, may your dilemma gain clarity as you continue to travel the path of *yama*.

Peace and beautiful practice.

Sincerely yours,

Nicole

CHAPTER 6

Probing Self-Consciousness:
How Do You Want to Be with Yourself?

"How many of us go to bed with a sense of accomplishment because we checked a lot of things off our task list or someone told us how "great" we were, or we "helped" others? What if we walked off stage altogether and put God there instead? Maybe then we could go to sleep at night, not with a sense of accomplishment, but with a sense of wonder, because all day we had been an attentive audience to the divine play. (9)"
— **Deborah Adele**

Winchester, MA—March 2, 2019

Dearest Yogini,

You and I number among the 36.7 million practitioners of yoga in the United States (as of 2016), up from 20.4 million in 2012. (12)

With so many conscious contenders within our ranks, it stands to reason that the industry that yoga has become is just as susceptible as any other enterprise to our capitalistic culture: The drive for financial gain, competition, and success. I have no intention of taking us down a rabbit hole of politics and persuasion; instead, I feel it is important to restate the need for each and every one of us to take ownership for the choices we make along the path of yoga, now more so than ever.

If we are not the forerunners of consciousness in this country, then perhaps we take on the responsibility to act well in the world (in accordance with *yama*) and to transmute self-preoccupation into self-awareness through our practice of *kriya yoga*, the 'yoga of action'. *Kriya yoga* is defined by Patañjali in *sutra II.1* as a composite of *tapas*, self-discipline with a quality of burning desire to burn away the impurities of body, senses, and mind; *svadhyaya*, the study of the teachings in order to know one's self; and *Ishvara praṇidhānā*, surrender of one's body, mind, and soul to some force greater than ourselves.

While *yama* teaches you to pay attention to your thoughts, to your inner dialogue and behaviors, *niyama* teaches you to take action to support the work of *yama*. Self-discipline, self-study, and sweet surrender are three of the five elements of *niyama*. The practice of *yama* is to pull back on the reins of our habitual conditioning and train the untamed mare of the mind how to be in the world. *Niyama* is a purification practice that allows the gem of your True Self, your spirit, to shine as brilliantly as it is meant to, free of anything and all that dulls and subjugates it.

And so, our wise guide Patañjali offers you the five tools of *niyama* to guide you in your evolution towards harmony with yourself and your life. *Niyama* allows you to continue your journey inward toward wholeness and discovering your destiny as the truth of who you are.

Saucha: Cultivate purity, to know your Self through simplicity and discernment so that your body, your thoughts, your emotions become clear reflections of you.
I have learned that to embody the heart of yoga you must first and foremost learn to respect and honor yourself. To this end, the wisdom practices of yoga teach you to become more resilient in the face of adversity, trauma, tragedy, threats, and other significant sources of stress—such as family and relationship problems, serious health problems, or workplace and financial stressors. In other words, by "tuning in" to yourself, you become more discerning around what "stuff" belongs to you and when someone else's vortex pulls you away from yourself. You learn to find an anchor within yourself, to bounce back from difficult experiences, and to love yourself unconditionally no matter what. This then becomes the practice of *saucha*.

It has taken me decades to realize that my self-talk sabotaged the way I perceived myself, judged myself, and treated myself. I know I am not alone in this. This could be an entire book unto itself, but would you not agree that we are entire generations of women (and men, transgender, etc.) who have learned from our respective social circles, our culture, and our families to believe we are insufficient, not enough, objects of sexual allure, material pleasures, or discarded commodities withering from neglect or abuse? We learn too quickly to disabuse ourselves of our inherent goodness and lovability.

This process of 'cleaning house' requires a big dollop of bravery, a good dose of respect, a dash of humor, and the absolute knowledge you are loveable, loving, and loved no matter anyone else's opinion of who you are or what you should do may be.

It can feel overwhelming to manage and feed the constant amount of effort and work that goes into keeping your world in a state of cleanliness, literally and figuratively. To start, it might take rather more energy to apply the quality of vigilance your situation may require to meet yourself in the right place. Yoga asks you to begin with 'cleaning' the body through diet and exercise—attention to the kind of fuel (quality of food) you put in your body and the practice of *asana*, or posture, the third and next step on the yogic path. And because the mind thinks thoughts that reflect ego-attachments to the material world, the mind too requires 'cleaning,' as it is more deeply enmeshed in the endless cycle of sensory pleasure and suffering.

Saucha of the mind is the practice of seeing, then ceasing and desisting with thoughts or emotions of (self) hatred, greed, pride, lust, envy, jealousy, etc. Once these improper habits are scrubbed clean—to the extent possible—from the slate of memory and conditioning, the original *sattvic*, or luminous, quality of the intellect shines forth, like a diamond, unclouded by such impurities.

This is joy. It's not that the habitual tendencies don't rear their ugly heads, but once recognized as such, the platitudes fade and your innermost light reflects back to you your own brilliance in the form of individuality, inspiration and ingenuity.

Santosa: Cultivate contentment by taking pause and noticing the spaces 'in between'.

This is courage! Keep up your travails and the burden of efforting shall subside. Our attention is always somewhere other than here; so notice, right now, *where is it, this attention of yours?* Connect with it and become curious about where it was and what it was doing (assessing, judging, criticizing, defending, analyzing, planning, etc.). Keep up your practice of mastering your senses: Of bringing the eyes back to inner focus; of listening in with the auditory faculties; of the taste buds savoring with savvy and discernment; of touching in upon the conditions of the body and qualities of the heart with kinesthetic sensitivity; of bringing the olfactory senses back to scent (scent is the sole sense capable of engaging us *uniquely* in the present moment).

And when you have gathered your senses and cultivated *eka-grata*, one-pointedness of the mind, when all your faculties become absorbed in this moment and no longer depend on external or mental stimulations, you have accessed *santosa*, contentment. This means that the next time an 'object of desire' (i.e. the beep or buzz of your phone) floats through the realm of your awareness, you catch yourself in the midst of any and all complicit tendencies, and restrain your senses from reaching out and embracing the desired reward. This practice requires a measure of dispassion so that, little by little, the object that craves your attention can be left alone without your need to reach for it. The vigilance and hard work you apply to your practice of catching yourself in the act of gratifying your craving softens with repetition until the day you arrive at the realization of its effortlessness. This means you can't think of a better place to be right now, embodied, and present. This, dear yogini, is your practice of *santosha*.

In yoga, *santosha* is ground for the absorbed state of *samadhi*, the eighth step or facet of the path of yoga, described by Patañjali (in *sutra III.3*) as your means to arriving at enlightened perception, a "fusion of the knower [you] and the process of knowing [intuitive wisdom] with the object to be known. (13)" How else might you define your state of 'enlightened perception', dear yogini? Your moving towards this state (of *samadhi*) with your practice of yoga—this movement towards seeing yourself more clearly—now extends to you the possibility of living right into clear resolution of your dilemma.

Tapas: Cultivate discipline with wisdom—Show up to do the work with sincerity and passion!

What are you passionate about dear yogini? What about your yoga sets you on fire? What makes you show up? I wish to know what fascinates you about your yoga! *Tapas* is the driver of passion and refers to the discipline it takes to show up and sustain your yoga, all the more in the face of hardship and challenge.

Personally, it is no longer the same passion for practice I once had when I first came to yoga that compels me to show up every day for my yoga; the practice is, after all, a practice: Some days I show up for it with ease, and others will take everything I have to not talk myself out of showing up in the way yoga asks me to. I have found every excuse in the book on the hardest days to not be with the dark and icky parts of myself, the parts that are vulnerable and insecure, the places that are tense or hold pain. Frankly, it is fearsome and, in some instances, downright insufferable.

Do I do this in solitude? Yes. You don't have to, but it is one way to see beyond the lies and mistruths we are subject to telling ourselves in order to get past the stuff we really don't want to see. The other way to see what needs to be seen is in relationship to someone who can hold you accountable or in whose presence you can see yourself more clearly. The passion for yoga reveals itself when you begin to experience the ways in which this practice sets you free.

The practice of *tapas* allows you, dear yogini, to burn through your own complicit consciousness and purify your conditioned reactivity to the people and events in your life that are certain to challenge your sense of what is valid (thinking, speech, behavior) and what isn't. You know that person—a boss, a parent, a former lover, a friend—who is subject to the same human condition as you or I. He hides his insufficiency behind the mantle of masculinity overcompensating with his alpha-ego or physical build, playing big by design thereby diminishing the 'other'. She shields her insecurity behind a façade of self-importance and maybe self-deprecating wit, seeking solidity and self-worth through actions that condescend to or belittle another's right to be. These patterns of conditioning are universal and laden with ruthless passive-aggression to match the pain and suffering on the backend. They make the perpetrator's ego-self feel better. And then there comes a time when what shows up for you feels less like anger or condemnation of the situation, and more like understanding and compassion for his suffering, for her pain. With determination and discipline, or *tapas*, you get to not participate in the theatrics and place yourself at a remove.

The Yogic Wisdom invites you to notice your emotional reactivity to these types of scenarios, to take a breath, a step back, then to zoom out and observe the whole mise en scène through a wide-angle lens. Notice the feeling that develops as a result of the conflict and respond with self-awareness and diplomacy, so to speak, to the offense in question. As yogis, you and I have the privilege of the practice and the possibilities of insight to perceive beyond the surface layer of such behaviors to an underlying dynamic that neither divides nor justifies but has the potential, always, to move each of us in the direction of harmony.

Tapas has the attribute of wisdom underlying its application to anything you do but especially your yoga, and allows you to sustain a consistent and dedicated practice without injury to yourself or others. This explains how you might bring the intelligence of *tapas* to your practice as a way of replacing old patterning with new habits while supporting the inward journey of the mind. What is the point of good practice, dear yogini, without the underlying friendliness (towards yourself and others) and the wisdom to be with what shows up?

When you embody the heart of yoga in the spaciousness of *upekshanam* or equanimous mind, so vast it can hold all of life's contradictions, you will notice that you are not disturbed by many of the things in your life that may once have sent you into a tailspin of reactivity, dejection, loneliness and depression—all states of relative impermanence, and the breath shows us this. (We will get to the power of the breath at a later time dear yogini).

Svadhyaya: Study, contemplate, retreat so that you may be guided to the seat of the Self.
Notice how your body feels, how your mind frames your experiences, and how you respond to the people, events, and circumstances in your life, and in this way, you begin to cultivate your ability to hear your inner voice of wisdom as it permeates the realm of your conditioned consciousness. Tuning into yourself is a way to bring you back to the place of your own heart so that you may live your life in truer fashion or at least as a truer reflection of you. This is the practice of *svadhyaya*.

Svadhyaya is all about getting to know yourself really well and perfecting the art of equanimity by seeing the space between a stimulus, or 'trigger', and your reactivity to it. Nowhere is this more apparent than in our triggered response to an event that recollects a previous trauma. Resilience in the face of adversity is not something you have or don't have. It involves behaviors, thoughts, and actions in adaptive and self-regulatory capacities that can be cultivated through the practice of getting to know yourself and through the breath.

It is not so much *what* needs to be done that is in question. Instead, notice how your mind dismisses, resists, rebels, or revolts against accepting or admitting the existence of a truth it does not want, or is too painful to see. Be vigilant in your own practice, dear yogini, as you notice any tendencies you may have towards dismissing that which keeps presenting itself to you in your practice as in your life. When denial is present, my experience is that life will find a way to throw adversity at you in a way you can no longer ignore. Should the path you find yourself on be ridden with obstacles, use the yogic wisdom to trust that another door, another way, will open up to you.

The responsibility to follow your path becomes a driving force as your yoga reveals itself to you in discrete increments and opens you up more and more to yourself. Use the tenets of yoga, *yama* and *niyama* alike, to be gentle and friendly towards yourself in the process of your evolution. We are too quick to subscribe to the thoughts, beliefs, and attitudes that will mislead us in our practice of yoga. When you rest in *svadhyaya*, studying yourself and your mental, intellectual, emotional, and physical predispositions, you can challenge the paradigms that present themselves to you. In this moment of seeing, you can shape-shift the context and texture of your thoughts to more accurately reflect how to be in alignment with what you want for yourself and how you wish to be in the world. Your dilemma may be a sticking point, so listen well to that within you which seeks to be heard. *Does the prospect of teaching yoga feel like a 'calling' or is it an ideal towards another end?*

Trust the trials and tribulations of time to serve as your guides should you wish to opt in to learning from them. I can reflect back on my once ardent desire to attend medical school (having applied three times) and recognize that, at each turn, all manner of excuses (in the guise of what was going on in my life at the time) persisted in holding me back from moving forward in that direction. By odd twists and turns of fate, I have discovered within my practice and teaching of yoga a holistic science of physical health and mental-emotional wellbeing that is far more suitable to my proclivity towards addressing the whole of a person rather than their disparate symptomatologies.

Get to know yourself, dear yogini, or in the language of yoga, practice *svadhyaya*. Insights and feelings arrive in all shapes and sizes and much of the time we miss them because we just aren't paying attention. Self-study is the practice of showing up again and again, tuning in to yourself, and seeking understanding through resources and persistent practice of the stuff that manifests in your awareness to always arrive back at yourself.

Isvara Pranidhana: And you move towards the Sacred Self, the light of universal consciousness.

It occurred to me as I was writing that I do not yet know your outlook on life. I have come to trust in its importance in how we approach life. My father was a driving force for the person I am today (and am still becoming) in the world. My brother and I would refer to our dad as the "optimistic pessimist." My father had an attraction to the more Shopenhauerian view of passion, irrationality, and pessimism as drivers for his sense of general discontent. My father, though, believed he had risen above it in a Nietzschean force-of-will such that his pessimism about the world in general was tempered by his optimism about his own position within that world. (14)

If you picked up this book, chances are you stand in the same strand of privilege as I. I am White (and while skin color should not separate us, it does my friend, and we must continue to strive for an un-coloring of cultures around the globe); I am a Woman; and I am a product of Western culture. The first 'coloring' affords me complicit anonymity from racial bias. The second means I am subject to the same patriarchy of those of my generation but because of the third I have access to a voice that I can make heard. I was born with certain privileges, such as education and a stable family life, many can only aspire to. And although my sight is compromised, I live in an able and intelligent body, and for this gift I am infinitely grateful. In other words, you and I hold a position in the world that *demands* that we take a stand and take action for the benefit of all humanity.

But first, the yogic wisdom informs us that, while our thoughts matter, they cannot be believed because they are subject to our conditioning, or *samskaras,* and the whims of our ego-self. They can, however, be controlled once perceived. This is our work through yoga. The whole first chapter of Patañjali's *Yoga Sūtras* is dedicated to describing the mind waves, or fluctuations of consciousness, to help the yoga practitioner to better understand and access the eight 'aids' and practices of ashtanga yoga. Your thoughts determine your speech, and your narratives determine your behaviors and the way you are in the world.

At first, the tenets of *yama* guide you to forego doing harm by directing your thoughts and communicating and acting with reverence and kindness (*ahimsa*); to dedicate yourself to the truth (*satya*); to refrain from desiring "more than" (*asteya*); to devote yourself to leading a balanced and harmonious life (*brahmacharya*); and to cultivate non-attachment to possessions and relationships in your life with awareness of the abundance that is already there (*aparigraha*).

Then, as the tenets of *niyama* instruct, you forego the attempt to strive and learn to respect, honor, and love yourself (*saucha*); only then can the awareness turn around and find that everything is there already (*santosa*); as you persist in your practice with the discipline and determination of *tapas,* this fire removes the distortions and impurities of your diamond-Self by burning through the toxicities of your complicit conditioning. This readiness for cultivating tolerance and knowing your very own truth is referred to in classical yoga as *svadhyaya,* the 'study of the self.' Finally, you arrive at the practice that cultivates the art of letting go and letting be, breath by breath, pose by pose, moment by moment; this is *Isvara pranidhana.*

In yoga, each neuronal impulse, every single cell and molecule of your being and all the fibers of your soul, are engaged towards this end—the surrender to something far vaster than the experience of our thinking faculty and the feelings of 'I'. It is to engage with the realm of quantum physics, to develop a faith that is born of your own experiences, and, ultimately, to trust in a supreme, universal, cosmic intelligence. Such release or movement towards the divine, states Patañjali (in *sutra II.45*) brings about the light of pure consciousness, revealing the radiance of the diamond of the True Self. Is this not the direction of your seeking? What else do you seek to see within yourself? Revel in these contemplations dear yogini. I bid you a good night and sound sleep!

Peace and beautiful practice.

Sincerely yours,

Nicole

CHAPTER 7

The Body's Prayer

"Don't move the way fear makes you move. Move the way love
makes you move. Move the way joy makes you move."
— **Osho**

Winchester, MA—March 3, 2019
Dear Yogini,

How many obstacles do you face every day that you somehow manage to survive and work through? I hope the proverbial 'putting out fires' is not an everyday occurrence for you. Yet it appears as more and more a part of our harrowed lives where emotions fray and tempers flare. Physical obstacles—like illness and injury—strike me as among the most challenging types. To not be of sound physical health or 'embodied', or to not be able to partake in the pleasures of being out in nature—walking, hiking, swimming, kayaking—would surely take away my joie de vivre. This then tends to make me more attached to positive outcomes as when my body feels stronger and more agile (so yes, I do love my *asana* practice!) and averse to being waylaid by sickness or physical impairment of any kind.

Asana is a practice of bringing all the elements that constitute our physical being—earth, water, fire, air and ether—into balance. Asana quite literally signifies the 'seat' upon which one sits or the manner in which one takes that seat, as in taking a 'posture'. This third facet of the eight-limbed path of yoga is established as the third 'indirect aid' to dissolving the impurities of the mind in order to bring about intuitive thinking, because it will bring you, the practitioner, up against nine impediments that show up in practice, described by Patañjali (in *yoga sutra I.30*) as (all shades of) illness, inertia, doubt, negligence/pride, idleness, sensual gratification, false perception, stagnation, and recidivism.

You have, and will continue to, come up against all of these in some form or another as obstructions to your personal progress and as distractions to your mind in asana. If you have 'suffered' the exertion of sustaining your concentration in the discerning muscular and energetic actions of a challenging warrior pose held for time, or the pockets of tension that arise when you are asked to feel into a yin pose, for example (typically a seated posture, sustained for time, at the edge of your comfort zone, with as little physical engagement as possible and with support as necessary to assist in disengaging muscular effort), you can conceive how the physical-sensory, emotional-energetic, and mental-spiritual impediments that come up for you in those instances can quickly deter you from your practice or further inform it. Practitioner's choice. But here's the gold nugget: When your consciousness is free from impediments, only then is self-realization possible, states Patañjali.

So ask yourself this, dear yogini: *In what ways is your personal practice progressing or stagnating?* Yoga, of course, is not built on philosophy alone. What I have come to value most about the path of yoga is the wisdom it proffers as a way to frame the conditions and experiences of life so as to minimize and reduce our reactivity to what shows up. Our human-ness, our foibles, and our flaws then become the substrate of our yoga practice and can serve as our best teachers if we can learn to see them, be with them, and act upon them with discernment rather than judgment, and with kindness rather than aggression.

I described for you in a previous letter how I lived in fear of cancer following my mother's diagnosis with non-Hodgkin's lymphoma. We all face fears of some adverse event befalling us or a loved one. These perceived threats to our existence stall us in our progress, putting us right up against the penultimate affliction, *abhinivesha*, the fear of death. Has this come up for you in practice dear yogini? You may have the advantage of an able body and a positive attitude to counter the effects of the years of wear-and-tear on the joints and the calamities of a broken heart. And still, you may well understand what it feels like to be limited by pain or incapacitated by some ailment, physical or emotional in nature. All of this then becomes a part of your yoga practice. It is when some event or circumstance of life feels impossibly hard that you notice that showing up for your practice becomes the challenge.

For me, this came in the form of a retinal detachment—two actually—at the grand age of 47. It is quite something to come up against the possibility of losing your sight, twice, and a whole other thing to be a front-row witness to the aftermath of a young daughter's tragic and sudden death. My boyfriend-at-the-time lost his 18-year old daughter and sole child in the blink of an eye, this impossible incident framed by my two retinal events. His greatest fear realized, there is no turning back the clock, no rewriting this story, no undoing his horrid irrevocable reality. I cannot say how he gets out of bed every morning. But he does. One foot in front of the other. I cannot judge his experience. I will not color the effect it has had on me, on us, with the narratives and stories my mind is prone to work with to try to make sense out of the nonsensical. And I won't call it perspective. My sight is imperfect at best yet seems prone to a particular consciousness: To see clearly things as they are. I still see the light and the light allows me to see. Over there, there is nothing but a finality to his 'gone-ness', an impossible darkness. And both are irrevocably true.

My practice has had to constantly shapeshift to meet the evolving requirements of eye surgery, recovery and healing; and then to support the space of a grief too profound to fathom. My physical practice looks nothing like it once did, but my yoga feels more intelligent, wiser, freer and more sincere. For now, I am learning to integrate all these sensitivities into my yoga practice as points of curiosity; without this inquisitiveness, I am as prone to dejection as the next person.

And to you I say, *How much to you want to pay the price—physically, emotionally, mentally, spiritually—of living and re-living in the present moment a narrative that is not yours?* You have inherited and adopted and no doubt played out stories you were told as a child or perhaps too, narratives you created in your head to make everything okay because that was all you could do at the time to make sense of the confusion, the hurt, the horror. On the one hand, *asana* might be practiced on the basis of unspoken assumptions around its intrinsic healing capacities; on the other hand, *asana* might be thought of as a means to prevent such unfortunate instances from occurring in the first place. But at the heart of *asana* practice lies the discerning quality of intelligence that weaves its way from how we engage our body in action to touching in upon the subtlest energetic effects of these actions. There is no hiding from or controlling the stuff of life as much as we may deceive ourselves into thinking we can. However, we can become more sophisticated in our reaction to and how we manage life's incidental liabilities and gross misfortunes when they do rear their heads, and more particularly when they reveal themselves in our body and pour forth onto our yoga mat. This is where the work of knowing yourself begins in earnest.

Asana, this third facet of Patañjali's ashtanga yoga and the physical aspect of your practice, can be used to hone your skills at inhabiting your body with more wisdom and sensitivity. *Asana* practice includes equal measures of persistent effort (*abhyasa*) to realize the objective of self-knowing and a corresponding release of attachment to the stuff that stands in the way (*vairagya*). (15) Do you get discouraged in practice? Bored by the sameness or rote repetition of postural sequencing? Easily distracted? *Abhyasa* reminds you to be fiercely focused and present to how you are engaging in practice and what you are engaging with, and so persistent effort builds on itself—the more you show up in practice, as in life, the more your practice and your path reveal themselves to you. *Vairagya* implies that consciousness is colored by all the things that have no measure of permanence—material objects, people, ideas, opinions, thoughts—and therefore also defines how we identify ourselves and relate to others. So the fluctuations of conscious are to be controlled through *abhyasa*, your persistence to show up for your practice, and *vairagya*, the mental strength you develop to overcome all obstacles to practice.

What attachments come up for you in your consciousness, dear yogini? What is it in your physical practice that stands in your way? Have you told yourself you are "too tight," "not flexible enough," "have no coordination," or do not have the right "body type" that makes you shy away from showing up? Perhaps your competitive or perfectionist drive pushes you towards an aggressive practice, or your proclivity for inertia towards intention to show up for practice minus the motivation. I have seen my own practice shift over time from an intense physicality to a milder physical practice. Whether I like it or not, my body is feeling the ailment of aging. So now my practice builds on endurance (holding poses for time) and being with the sensitivities of my body with more discrimination in each posture and with my mind at attention.

In *sutras I.21 and I.22*, Patañjali emphasizes the critical importance of the strength of our 'desire' in determining how easily we will attain our goal of attaining victory over the mind. It also determines how well you will overcome obstacles when they arise, in practice as in life, and indicates what kind of yoga aspirant you are. The aspirant you are in yoga is not a given; it must be earned. This means that, no matter what, keep showing up. Over the course of our lives, we will all vacillate between three levels of aspiration in practice where the mildest degree of desire can be neutralized by fear of failure, the spark of motivation too subtle; the moderate aspirant starts their quest with great enthusiasm but drops into disappointment or denial when confronted with obstacles in practice; and then there is an intense burning desire that consumes all other desires and the deterrents of practice, although burnout is a potential risk to those with such an enthusiastic drive.

There was a time I strived for perfection in practice. The dancer in me, the 'good daughter', the 'people-pleaser' sought to avoid conflict at all costs. I began my practice of yoga with the intense fire of desire that burned through all initial obstacles because I was fighting my mother's cancer, my father's death and a plethora of other unconscious conditions, including, 'though I couldn't 'see' it yet, the demise of my marriage. And then life taught me to slow down, and not always gently. Whether you strive for standards of external accomplishment, or listen to the 'shoulds' and the 'cannots' decided by your ever-fickle mind, or quash the traumas and tragedies of the heart that have taken up residence in your body and are stored in your subconscious, all of it bubbles up at the end of the day.

If it does not show up on your yoga mat, then it will show up in your life. So perhaps it is not such a bad thing if you can take the seat of *asana* and 'act' upon your body with wisdom. Notice the distractions, the discouragements, and the boredom that are inevitable components of practice, and allow those unprocessed narratives and emotions behind them to rise up and occasionally disturb the smooth surface level of pretense that protects your inner realm. You don't have to know where these sensitivities come from or what they represent. The yogic wisdom asks that you simply notice them as they arise in your awareness, acknowledge and feel into them in your body, and then discern how your practice shifts as a result of placing your attention on the stuff that shows up.

On your mat, you follow a directive in class, and although you conceptually grasp the action or intelligence behind it, it makes no sense to you in this moment. There is no signal from brain to body. In fact, it may feel like it is in direct opposition to what your body wants to do or everything you think you know. As the directive permeates your consciousness, notice the chatter: *"No way. I'm not doing that!"* shrieks the Fear. *"That doesn't feel right,"* grumbles the Body. *"Why on earth would I do that?"* sneers the Skeptic. *"I don't think so. I won't, I can't. I'm not [good, able, competent, thin] enough,"* whispers the voice inside your head, which you barely hear, but it is sufficient to shut you down to your experience.

And then, with some passage of time, you are back on your mat once again for your *asana* practice. The inner narratives are too slow on the uptake today, and something else happens. I know this to be true from my own experience and as feedback from way too many practitioners to not believe its inherent value: Your body's innate intelligence bypasses your brain. Your somatic body automatically processes what the instructional directive is implying without going through the machinations of your thoughts that hinder and obstruct the flow of information and insight. I call these instances "moments of *samadhi*," or brief flashes of insight and absorption that amount to a mini-moment of enlightenment where the brain and the body sync up in agreement.

I can't tell you exactly how this feels to you in your body and in your experience of the posture once arrived at, but the practical contact with *asana* itself offers up the dual qualities of steadiness in action infused with 'sweetness' or 'ease'. Patañjali describes these postural textures as *sthira* and *sukha* respectively, in *sutra II.46—sthira sukham āsanam,* his singular description of asana itself out of this entire collection of sutras. When your body arrives at the harmonious blend of strength and softness in postural practice, "steadiness of intelligence and benevolence of spirit, (16)" then you have, in essence, "taken your seat."

In my experience, this dichotomous essence of *asana* permeates my way of being in the world, steadfast and grounded on the inside while fluid and adaptable on the outside as I begin to trust in my own experience and in myself.

Patience and persistent practice, dear yogini; the fruits of your efforts will continue to reveal themselves in their own time and space. This is a promise.

Sincerely yours,

Nicole

CHAPTER 8

Balancing Prana

"I took a deep breath and listened to the
old bray of my heart: I am, I am, I am."
– **Sylvia Plath**

Winchester, MA—March 20, 2019

Dear Yogini,

Welcome to this day! With the advent of the vernal equinox and the lengthening light of day, one can feel the clarity and freshness in the air and the birdsong carried by the breeze bringing us out of our New England winter and officiating our season of spring. It is also my father's birthday today, so I take precious moments to simply breathe and savor my breath and to rest in gentle remembrance of him and the memories that bring me joy. He gave me the gift of independence; and yoga, my love language, has guided me towards the intimacy of how to be unconditionally loving towards myself without concern for what anyone else thinks of me. Breathing in, I claim my independence, my sense of Self; breathing out, I settle into the familiarity of me and the confidence I gain by being friendly with myself.

This intentional modulation of the breath, or breath control, is *prānāyāma*, the fourth and pivotal facet of your practice. Breath is our life force and allows us to meet each moment with awareness. It is your guide in yoga and reflects too your state of being. Do you notice your breath getting quicker with anticipation when you wait uncertainly for what comes next, or for the other shoe to drop? Are you aware of how you hold your breath when you are deep in concentration? Or the exertion of your exhale when you are putting extra physical effort into something, let's say your postures? Do you notice that your breath becomes shallower with trepidation? Can you feel when you forget to breathe *in*? Can you touch with your awareness that moment you notice you haven't been breathing at all?

And here it is that our energy, our prana, is derived from our breathing. Take a deep breath and notice the pause it gives you to come back to the present and savor the moment. When we don't breathe well, we become depleted and wonder at our lethargy, our sluggishness, our insomniac tendencies, our inability to focus and concentrate—the litany of ailments and impediments to our well-being. Herein lies the brilliance of yoga: The breath, while automatic, stands alone as the only subsystem the conscious mind can put into 'manual override.' So it is through conscious manipulation of the movements of the breath that we can recalibrate our entire system. In other words, you and I have the ability to control the following characteristics of the breath:

1. Its directionality: We can draw the breath in (descending) and move the breath out (ascending).

2. Its hyper-dimensionality: We can gauge the intrinsic capacity of the breath to expand in all directions, like the rays of the sun.

3. Its depth and duration: We can stretch the breath out to make it deeper and slower as with the practice of the oceanic *ujjayi pranayama*, or victorious breath; we can shorten the breath to quicken it and make it shallower (as in hyperventilation, or with the practice of *kapalabhati pranayama*, 'skull-shining' breath, where the emphasis is placed on the exhalation of the breath).

What the yogic wisdom understood about the breath long before the science corroborated its capacity to directly regulate the autonomic nervous system is that how we breathe has a direct influence on our automatic physiological responses and thus emotional reactivity and behaviors. More specifically, breath control—with particular attention to slowing the breath and deepening the breath—helps to increase vagal tone which means you can respond to stress in a more measured and resourced fashion.

With mindfulness and consistency, *pranayama*, combined with other yoga techniques and practices, empowers us to increase our window of tolerance and resilience to traumatic or stressful events. First, you develop awareness of your individual reactions to situations, and then, using the tools and techniques of *pranayama* or restorative yoga practices, you can monitor your reactivity to external stimuli and gain control over your own behavior, emotions, and thoughts. This is self-regulation and personal agency. In yoga, this quality of sustained psychological stability of mind through a range of experiences and situations, including those of conflict and change, is *upekshanam*, or equanimity, a concept I introduced you to in one of my previous letters.

Come back to that very first tenet and aid to your yoga, *yama*, the conduct that is practiced in the form of restraining your natural tendencies towards unbecoming behavior or actions that do not serve your best interest. And now consider its foremost principle, *ahimsa,* respect for all living things (nonviolence). Ask yourself this: Can I forego doing harm to myself (by what I put in my body and how I treat myself) and unto others (by the way I behave and treat them) by directing my thoughts, and communicating and acting with reverence and kindness? The breath is your guide as you persevere at your practice, dear yogini. For each step forward, there may be two, three, five steps back. But the breath is your constant companion. Turn towards it, and invite it in. It is your life force and at times may well feel like a lifeline. Grab ahold of it, and let it serve as a tether when you are frayed, distraught, or brokenhearted.

How many times a day do we forget to breathe? And yet the day marches on as does life, without regard for whether we are keeping up with it or not. With all the yoga in the world you wonder perhaps at your ability to stay true to the practice, dear yogini. I say this: Keep breathing. Yoga is not a perfect process because we are not perfect in our approach to life. But it is a process nonetheless, and the breath shows us this. The breath does not stop of its own accord until the final exhale, so it behooves us to ride the waves of the breath and with it the rising and falling away of each moment's experiences.

The breath asks us to honor what it is to be 'simply human', this common condition from which no one is exempt. How many times have I fallen off my practice wagon, have I failed to 'achieve' my idea of what is 'right' or 'wrong,' what is 'good behavior' and what is 'bad behavior'? Better yet, what happens when I make it personal? *I suck at this* [by whose standards of excellence? I ask you]. *I'm not good enough* [for whom?]. *I'm a disappointment* [to whom?]. *I'm a (complete and absolute) failure* [in what regard?].

I hope, dear yogini, this is not part of your self-talk, that you do not berate yourself and bring yourself down, in practice, of your own accord. But, if you do—and we have all done so at some time or another—know simply to bring your attention to this too. When I give myself permission to pause, to take a deep breath and savor the moment, I see that filament of thought, that sensate expression for what it is. It is only that someone, somewhere, at some point in my life disparaged me or invalidated my sense of self. I ascribed it significance, embodied it, then began to believe it, and it became my truth. The awareness I have cultivated through *pranayama* in combination with my yoga has served to shift the dynamic of my thinking and how I speak to myself and to my body in *asana*, in prayer. In essence, I have learned to repattern my perception. (17) Is it not worth persevering in practice to shift the dynamic of our understanding, our beliefs, and deepest truths towards manifesting the things we desire for ourselves and in the world?

Nothing is sustainable without breath. Your in-breath is your source of *prana*, the vital principle (in contrast to the vital air that arises in the thoracic cavity, *prana vayu*). In yoga, the breath is both the most essential and most crucial component of practice because it subdues the 'monkey mind' and anchors the attention so you can direct awareness and the energy of your thinking to where you want it to go. It is the connector, the bridge between brain and body, mind and matter, spirit and soma. Your breath is the *brahma sutra*, this thread of consciousness that defines the current of Life Force (or *prana*) by which all of the universal objects are bound together. Your breath brings this light of awareness and the discerning capacity of the intellect into the realm of the physical—into your body, into your practice and right into *asana* and perceived bodily sensations. Your breath-based interventions restore and enhance your ability to feel and be more and more at ease with your somatic experiences. So you can see how the breath is a powerful force for shifting dynamics within the body as well as within the mind and our thinking. It becomes a key ingredient to then shifting our speech and behaviors in truth towards serving our own highest good.

Pranayama is the combination of two concepts we are now familiar with—*prana*, vital life force; and *yama*, holding back, restraint. You breathe, you pay attention to your breath, and you modulate your breath with *pranayama* techniques to remember to be intensely present to what you are doing and how you feel in the moment. *Pranayama* brings all physiological systems into balance and into synergy one with the other. And because your consciousness is colored by your attachments to sense objects—whether your environment, other people, your thoughts, ideas, opinions, narratives—your breath serves to control your senses by drawing them inwards to focus on the subtlest movements of *prana* under the surface-layer of awareness. I leave you in the sensate arms of Spring to contemplate this.

Practice with patience, breathe deeply, sleep soundly.

Sincerely yours,

Nicole

CHAPTER 9

Taming the Senses

"Pratyahara... The movement of the mind
toward silence rather than toward things."
— **Donna Farhi**

Winchester, MA—March 25, 2019

Dear Yogini,

Withdrawing from the world is not so challenging for the introvert in me personally. What I find more provocative is removing my attention from the constant deluge of information and swarm of online activity which test my patience and lead me to adopt an all-or-nothing sort of approach to dealing with it! How do you manage this in your life dear yogini? I have found that resisting this sensory and digital overload is of little use as it just seems to invite more of the same.

The practice of what yoga calls *pratyahara*, retiring the senses, serves in a powerful way to manage the uncontrollable stream of data that makes its way to us. Instead of getting pulled towards these myriad sources of distraction (which have a tendency to make me feel anxious and ungrounded), *pratyahara* allows us to shift our senses, and thereby our attention, inwards. In this practice, my feelings of nervousness begin to dissipate, and I become a little more anchored in the solidity of my physical being and the steadfastness of self.

Your commitment to the process of noticing your breath and becoming aware of your breathing with all its subtle and not so subtle inflections is commendable. Your dedication to your yoga will enable you to attend to the ebb and flow of the sensations and experiences that arise and fall away with each breath. The breath not only draws the light of your awareness to your body; it also has the capacity to quite captivate your sensing organs—eyes, ears, nose, skin, and tongue. Each of these, in turn, is associated with a particular sensory sensibility—to see, to hear, to smell, to touch, to taste. Meanwhile, your senses continuously and incessantly draw raw information from the reality you are experiencing in this moment, as the mind, in its thinking capacity, is always thinking. They send this constant stream of information to the brain for framing (labeling), understanding (that is, conceptualizing based on your personal experiences to date), analyzing (what you decide to do with this raw data), and determination (how you 'package' this information for use further down the line).

So now, we move into the realm of the subtle energy body and *pratyahara*. You now ask your senses to turn their focus away from that which exists outside ourselves: The seeking of gustatory, olfactory, auditory, tactile, and predominantly visual satisfaction (as in our use of devices, or the ways in which we measure ourselves up against others, engage gossip, spread rumors, etc.); and the getting caught up in the stories that the mind contrives to make sense of, gain excitement from or avoid the painful parts of life and living.

As you engage with this practice of retiring your senses from the world outside yourself, you invite the possibility of finally sitting with your felt-sense, the way you actually *feel* on the inside. Take your gut instinct for example; if we could feel its energy and understand its significance in the moment of its manifestation, we wouldn't need to put all that mental "figuring out" energy into overriding the discomfort it creates within us. When this energy has an underlying temperament of fear, uncertainty, distress, or the unfamiliar, it is common to shut ourselves down to it. What energy we do have is expended resisting these feelings, pushing them away, denying them, and finally packing them up in metaphorical boxes that we shove into attic-recesses of the brain or into basement storage within our cells and tissues. It takes a whole bunch of energy to store and hold onto all those unwanted expressions of who we have come to believe we are at our core or who we think we should be in the eyes of others.

Dear yogini, do you ever feel like you are not an entirely true reflection of who you want to be or know yourself to be in your universe, teacher of yoga or not? Allow the yogic process to reveal its wisdom to you as you march forward in practice, and trust that you shall live into the answers to your question and the questions to come you have not yet asked! The more you are able to practice *pratyahara* as a common occurrence, the more you are then able to catch yourself in the midst of your own reactivity.

Over time, you begin to perceive and feel into the ways in which you come into conflict with yourself, its external expression polarizing the situation with blame and shame, he said/she said, wrong and right, good and bad, not guilty, guilty: *I really want to attend this yoga festival! But I really need to be home for the kids.* Guilt is polarizing like this, the no-win situation, such a perfect opportunity to tune in and ask which truth feels more right in this moment.

In the Eastern perspective, or the *Pancha Koshas* (five sheaths) model, on health and well-being, the vagus nerve (18) essentially serves as a bridge between our gross bodies (the outer-lying, most general, physical sheath, *annamaya kosha*) and our subtle energy bodies (the underlying permeating sheath of *pranamaya kosha*). The vagus nerve acts as a central 'switchboard' between the central nervous system (which includes the central processor, the brain, and the spine) and the autonomic nervous system (which controls the involuntary functions of the body, such as heartbeat, digestion, sex drive, and breathing), essentially connecting our conscious and unconscious minds. This may well be of the utmost relevance to our overall well-being because our yogic practices have the capacity to powerfully effect the vagus nerve and therefore, quite literally, our peace of mind and happiness (or lessening of our suffering). In yoga, this subtle nerve plexus is called *kurma nadi,* named for the turtle who withdraws his head into his shell when threatened or agitated. When energy moves through *kurma nadi*, all systems are subdued and the mind becomes quiet.

I find it fascinating that some ninety percent of the nerve fibers of the enteric nervous system (our gut) run one-way from the ganglionic mass (plexus) of nerves in the belly (above the navel, below the base of your sternum), commonly known as the Solar Plexus, via the vagus nerve up to the brain. It is not for nothing that our enteric nervous system is referred to more and more as our 'second brain.' When your gut feeling travels from the gut to your higher brain at the moment of its showing up in your overarching awareness, the 'light of consciousness' allows you to bypass or categorically override your instinctual response or reactivity to the situation. That's a pretty intricate system we have at our disposal. Isn't this worth knowing more about?!

The enteric nervous system executes most of our everyday tasks once they become second nature, or habitual. This explains then why the more repetitive tasks, like the practice of *asana,* or the synergy of breath and movement known as *vinyasa,* shift from originating in our conscious (or 'thinking' mind) as newcomers to yoga to happening in our subconscious (gut) when we become more adept at the practice. It would take far too much of our brain's capacity to have to focus on every small aspect of the tasks of yoga over and over and over again. Instead, they get handed over to our autonomic (automatic) background systems, and the consciousness is then free to apply more and more the qualities of discrimination and discernment to how we engage with our practice and, by extension, our lives. Until such a time as we arrive at unwavering experiential knowledge which illuminates truth and non-truth, fact and fiction, real and imaginary and leaves no room for doubt. This is, according to Patañjali, *viveka-khyati.* (19)

And so, to change or shift the dynamic of habitual behaviors or conditioned responses—positive or negative—you must engage the motherboard of the brain to prompt change and to inspire re-patterning of undesirable habits in the direction of more desirable patterns of thought, speech and action. This capacity for your brain (like your muscles) to repattern with repetition and frequency over time (and thus reorganize itself by forming new neural connections throughout life) is the science of neuroplasticity and is a built-in effect of the yogic process.

When you begin to touch into your physical body and allow yourself to *be* with the primordial and conditioned sensate experiences that arise from your gut feelings, you engage a process known as self-regulation which cultivates resilience. Resilience is the ability to bounce back from stressful or traumatic events with less and less reactivity. Your yoga empowers you, dear yogini, to discover yourself to be a greater person by far than you ever dreamed yourself to be.

Pratyahara strengthens your emotional intelligence. It is the way your sense perceptions shine upon your conditioned mental impressions, recollections, and psychological imprints. This collective conditioning is known in yoga as *samskara*. You have come across this concept in relation to *yama*, you may recall. In order to see ourselves more clearly in relationship to others we need to perceive, get to know and understand our patterns of reactivity, our *samskaras*. I urge you to get to know them well, dear yogini, for you are in constant relationship with your *samskaras* throughout your practice.

The energy that drives your emotions gains or loses significance and momentum based on how your rational mind understands and interprets the barrage of information that comes its way. This then has the potential to pave the way for the six "poisons:" anger, lust, greed, desire, pride, and envy. Also known as the six passions (for the fiery, or *rajasic*, quality driving them), these 'enemies of spiritual practice' come up all the time for anyone who is remotely human, with more energy driving some of these states and less underlying others. These states can quite literally suck you into their energetic vortex as the funnel cloud of a cyclone rotating all manner of dust and debris beneath it. This we call drama!

In practice, you will tend towards avoiding pain and gravitate towards all things pleasurable, unable to hold the space between stimulation and response. Your consciousness provides greater discernment, perceiving the energy as energy, without judgment and without being consumed by it. In a*sana*, you can apply the practice of *pratyahara* to discerning the sensory 'edges' of a posture or movement: Do I need to apply restraint to my actions (which may be true for a practitioner who inhabits a 'flexible' or hyperarticulate body)? Or conversely (if my body is tight or restricted by injury), can I soften my effort? Does my body feel safe here? Does it feel held? Does it feel loved?

The more you practice *pratyahara*, the more you will be able to catch yourself in the midst of your own sensate experiences and reactivity to what is. Honor the things you need to do for yourself. Learn to trust yourself through the wisdom of your experiences so you can hold safe space for yourself not just in practice but at all times. Come back to your practice of *asteya*, the third yama or restraint, dear yogini. Do not rob yourself of your own valuable sensory experiences by comparing yourself outwardly to anyone else. Here, the poet Galway Kinnell reminds us of our own brilliance:

> *"Though sometimes it is necessary*
> *to reteach a thing its loveliness,*
> *to put a hand on its brow*
> *of the flower*
> *and retell it in words and in touch*
> *it is lovely*
> *until it flowers again from within, of self-blessing"*
> **–Galway Kinnell** (20)

Make way then for *pratyahara*. Become familiar with your feelings and your passions so their qualification becomes the substrate of your practice. Withdraw into yourself like a caterpillar into her cocoon. Unlike the intellect which operates along the lines of reasoning, your sensate understanding moves from looking out to seeing in, from outer listening to inner hearing. Your head is where all your sense organs abide (although the skin covers your body's entire surface to protect from damage or harm), so draw your metaphorical turtle head inside its shell, retreat to the sanctuary of your heart, tune into that quiet voice, the kinesthetic sensitivity in the deepest layers of your being that serves you in your valiant quest for an answer.

Somewhere, in one of those metaphysical boxes you stashed away a long while back, lies the solution to your dilemma dear yogini. Go exploring. Venture forward! Use the safe sanctum of *pratyahara* practice to become curious about what lies within. As the caterpillar undergoes the process of metamorphosis, the energy freed up from your practices of being with yourself and feeling your feelings allows you to take flight in the direction of your dilemma unfolding, as a teacher or not as a teacher of yoga, but certainly as a beautiful butterfly.

Peace and patient *pratyahara* practice.

Sincerely yours,

Nicole

CHAPTER 10

Gathering the Mind

"I have been a seeker and I still am, but I stopped asking the
books and the stars. I started listening to the teaching of my Soul."
— **Rumi**

Monday, March 30, 2019

Dear Yogini,

Like the lotus to the sun, your soul is always reaching for the light to meet itself in truth. Throughout this process there are periods of darkness and moments you will be called to rest right where you are. It is a natural cycle and has an innate rhythm unique to your be-ing. *Dharana* is a state of mind in single-pointed concentration that unfolds from drawing in of the senses in *pratyahara*. It is the sixth facet of the yogic path, and the first direct aid to perceiving your true Self; in the

95

first *sutra* of Book III of *The Yoga Sūtras*, Patañjali describes *dharana* as the gathering of consciousness to focus it within.

You retire your senses as the lotus flower closes in upon itself and retreats to the dark cool just below the water's surface once the sun retires. You gather your attention to the gentle coming and going of your breath. It is said that flowers that tuck themselves in for the night aren't sleepy; they are just highly evolved: The bottom-most petals of these flowers grow at a faster rate than the upper-most petals and thus coerce the flowers to shut, possibly a protective mechanism or a way to conserve energy (or odor) for the daytime when pollinating insects are most active. Perhaps you too, at rest in quiet concentration, are preserving your energy for when the outside world assaults you with its busyness and bustle.

You are transitioning, dear yogini, from the realm of practice, per se, to progressive internal states that evolve from your continuous application of the earlier facets of the Yogic Wisdom. *Pratyahara* begins the rather arduous (if I may say so) task of becoming familiar with your internal states and how they make you feel. With *dharana*, states Patañjali, you sit and begin to work on the various qualities of the mind, or *gunas*, and their energetic manifestation as *vrittis*, oscillations of thoughts like the repetitive motion of sine-waves.

The three primary qualities of the mind are a reflection of nature, or cosmic intelligence (known as *prakriti* in the language of the *sūtras*) which consists of energy, matter, and consciousness: (21) *Sattva guna* is defined by luminosity and brilliance; *rajas guna* by action, motion, and passion; and *tamas guna* by inertia, density, and darkness. According to this worldview, the *gunas* have always been and continue to be present as dynamic forces of influence and change in all things in the world, including your consciousness and mine.

As an aspect of cosmic intelligence, our consciousness is subject to the influence of these vacillating qualities, these *gunas* that inform our (five) states of mind:

- The mind may be dull and ignorant, *tamas guna* driving it towards inertia and listlessness, as when we are engrossed in television.
- The mind may be in a state of neglect or distraction when we become too ensconced in our devices (*tamas* and *rajas gunas* at play).
- The mind becomes restless, hyperactive, or agitated under the influence of *rajas guna*, when we are overwhelmed by our 'to-do' lists, anxious and stressed.
- The mind becomes single-pointed, focused, and attentive when *sattva guna* predominates.
- The mind is restrained, controlled, and achieves *nirodha* with the suspension of all thought; here, all three *gunas* are dissolved.

This ultimate state of mind, *nirodha*, is characterized by the suspension of the thought-waves of the mind (22) (in order to see one's True Self clearly). This then becomes the foundation for your next assignment dear yogini, the seventh facet, *dhyana*, the art of meditation.

With peace and ever more concentration in practice.

Sincerely,

Nicole

CHAPTER 11

Consciousness

"The thing about meditation is: You become more and more you."
– David Lynch

Concord, MA—April 2, 2019

Dear Yogini,

Meditation, *dharana*, is like your silent footfall upon the warm sifting of sand, your thoughts, grains of multicolored sand on the mandala of the mind, your attention alighting briefly, without regard. The mind is neither completely still nor empty of thought; it is just that you have become more adept over time and with practice at sinking beneath the habitual ripples of thought, the *vrittis*, to settle into the safe sanctuary of stillness within yourself where peace lies.

I came to meditation by way of a random compact disc and the sound of Jack Kornfield's voice and gentle humor. The narration and brief meditative exercises softened the sorrow that sat in my heart after my father passed away, I would sit on my yoga mat and wonder where the energy was going to come from to engage my *asana* practice. I just sat and sat and sat. In essence, without realizing this at the time, I was sitting with my grief, with a sense of despair in the world.

My father's memorial was held in Geneva, Switzerland (where I spent my adolescence). It would have been his 68th birthday—March 20th, 2003—the day a United States-led coalition of countries invaded Iraq (in breach of International Law) as part of a declared war against international terrorism and its sponsors, notably Al-Qaeda, following the terrorist attacks on September 11, 2001. While the administration of U.S. President George W. Bush declared war on Saddam Hussein contending that the Iraqi government was in the process of developing (or had developed) chemical weapons and weapons of mass destruction, I stood in front of a sea of bodies and faces reading my posthumous letter to my father: *"Dear Daddy..."* Tears streaming, sobs caught in my congested throat, I gasped between words to catch my breath with the sincere hope he could hear me and know how many lives he had touched with his universally agreed-upon larger-than-life presence and generosity of spirit.

The mass of folk from all over the world—a testament to my father's combined intention to befriend pretty much everyone he met and his lifelong plan to visit every country on the face of the planet (which he came pretty close to judging from the reams of paper in each of his multitude of passports)—spilled outside the physical bounds of the (Presbyterian) Church of Scotland. This Kirk stood near the hotel where we celebrated his life to the catchy beats of ABBA (his request) and in the company of family, his colleagues, and myriad friends.

I remember, on this beautiful Spring day, standing alone at the balustrade dressed in my purple—color of consciousness—cocktail dress, gazing out at the scintillating Lac Léman and Geneva's most famous landmark, the Jet d'Eau, and contemplating the dichotomy between the peace of this singular moment in time and the shock-and-awe bombing campaign I understood to have just started in Iraq. Somewhere in that brief solitary moment the sounds around me faded, I saw nothing but the blue of the sky, a soft warmth pervaded my whole being, and I knew myself to be connected through some magic to the glory and spirit of my father or something vaster still that made me feel okay.

This was my first conscious understanding of meditation. I recollect many instances of absorption as a child and, given my proclivity to introversion and solitary pursuits from childhood to the present, this was perhaps more obvious to me than it might have been to most. Do you remember, dear yogini, when and why meditation became a part of your practice, if it is indeed something you practice, even sporadically? I once thought meditation to be the sort of practice that "other people" did. To be honest, I was a little above it at the time, which I'll gladly attribute to my youth partnered with ignorance.

It's ironic to hear folks explaining why meditation is <u>not</u> for them: "I can't sit still and you want me to, *what?*" or "My mind is way too busy for that!" What better place to start a practice of meditation than with a busy mind! Of course, just the idea of sitting is an impractical impossibility if your body is restless and constantly seeking sensation or movement as distraction, which explains why Patañjali introduces your postural practice, or *asana*, as the third facet of practice, well before this monster of meditation. Your breath, remember, reflects your state of mind and has the singular capacity to influence the vagus nerve and the parasympathetic relaxation response, so attending to the breath, with the practice of *pranayama* to harmonize your nervous system, is advocated to precede the art of sitting for meditation.

Then there are your senses, a serious source of distraction given that your eyes, ears, nose, tongue, skin, and gut are constantly at play with the reality around you, and more and more devoted to seeking gratification outside of yourself. Do you notice how your attention gets swallowed up in the disturbing vortex of an accident on the highway or the gripping content of a reality show on television (or in the news), how you can become so entangled in someone else's trauma or tragedy or caught up in the excitement of your adrenaline-laden virtual Amazon expeditions, only to become aware of being aware of how beholden you are to these distractions that are in actuality taking place outside of your immediate experience and separating you from yourself?

The same attention and awareness that brings you back from the brink of these sensory sinkholes—the practice of *pratyahara*—are also present in *dharana* (contemplation) and brought to *dhyana*, or meditation, the seventh facet of our yogic path, as too to the initial states of *samadhi*. For most of us mere mortals, *samadhi* will be experienced as ephemeral moments of self-absorption—when we perceive the phenomenon of light's spectrum in the rainbow after the storm, pause at day's dawning to absorb the magic of the moment, appreciate the serendipitous encounters and coincidental contrivances of the universe at play, where, in that instant, we gain an understanding of what it is to feel 'connected,' at one with all, and at peace with one's self.

Meditation, you see, is just the very simple practice of 'plugging in.' What is not so simple, and frankly quite daunting at times because of the plethora of obstacles, hindrances, and *samskaras* (conditioned patterns of perception and reactivity), is the sitting and being with the fickleness of the body and the mind. Meditation practice is really not *not* an option, not in this day and age of sensory overwhelm and soul deprivation. This idea is corroborated by the overused concept of "mindfulness" and purveyor of meditation in our present culture. You can spend a lot of money trying to figure out how to meditate, when to meditate, where to meditate, and how long to meditate for. The same holds true for yoga too, an industry which has grown by leaps and bounds in the last decade alone. There are such copious quantities of audiovisual, digital, online and the usual traditional resources nowadays, for yoga and meditation alike, that it is your responsibility, dear yogini, to be judicious in picking your sources of knowledge and any programming and training you choose to engage in. And while there are many platforms for practice, there appear to be fewer hours in the day and less-to-no space in our calendars in which to pursue our loftier intentions. And of course, do not neglect to attend to the resistances that reveal themselves to you in meditation; these are "truth-indicators" that help to guide you away from the resistance in the direction of meeting your own needs. Relish those quiet serendipitous moments when inspiration or insight arises in your consciousness and remember them when you may need them the most.

May you have a magical meditation experience.

Sincerely yours,

Nicole

CHAPTER 12

Simply Being

*"As a naturally pure crystal appears to take the color of everything
around it yet remains unchanged, the yogi's heart remains pure
and unaffected by its surroundings while attaining a state of
oneness with all. This is Samādhi. (23)"*
– **Nischala Joy Devi** *[Yoga Sutra I.41]*

Winchester, MA—April 4, 2019

Dear Yogini,

I have derived so much real-life benefit from yoga that I only share
my experiences and my understanding of the science and methodology
of yoga to demonstrate its transformative effects. I hold the candid belief
that no matter how life shows up for you, your sincere embodiment
of the essence of yoga will serve you in all regards and, in particular,
in living into an answer to your question. Eventually, dearest yogini,

your resolute and vigilant enterprise on the yoga mat will lead you to a clear resolution of your dilemma for the simple reason you will become clear on your thoughts rather than identify with them in mistaken or confused understanding. You will touch the heart of your true self that has the clarity of a "transparent jewel." (24)

When you understand and see for yourself the cyclical nature of your conditioning, you may then choose to release yourself of those beliefs and so-called friendships that no longer serve your self-evolution. The time to do so is when you notice your resistance to what is. And as you continue to unburden yourself from the weight of your stories, narratives, relationships and *samskaras* that are now obsolete your consciousness expands and you reflect your truth as a diamond its radiance.

Thus, *samadhi* is experienced as the state of resting in your own clarity, in your own truth. This is what is meant by the "light of the True Self." For most of us, *samadhi* reveals itself in those subtlest of moments of inattention to our outside reality and inner thinking. Eventually perhaps, total absorption is achieved—this ability to rest in *purusha*, the 'witness', and step into the power of perceiving reality as it is, where the coverings, deceptions, illusions, and contraptions of the mind fall away and the light of consciousness shines through.

I am not suggesting that you read *The Yoga Sūtras of Patañjali* for leisure, but it is helpful to understand where to go looking for the sources to your questions as they come up in your yoga experiences, and they will. It is in *sutra I.15* that you will find the first of eight instances of the word *"samādhi"* in the Yogic Wisdom. Here, its meaning can be better understood by knowing its derivation and the context in which it is used. It comes from the stem *"ādhi,"* meaning to think on, reflect, contemplate, or hold in mind. The prefix *"ā"* here indicates comprehensiveness or all-inclusiveness, reaching up to and including a certain limit. The prefix *"sam"* means collected together, or it expresses a quality of completeness, (25) as to abide in the unity of the mind, and rest within Self in a state of "oneness."

Samadhi is not an advanced or mystical state of consciousness in its more common or misappropriated usage. It is rather more simply stated as a 'coming home' to the Self, or a belief in the purity of your spirit. Can you see how every other facet of the eight-limbed path is a pre-requisite for this experience? *Samadhi* is not a state to be achieved, for there is nothing to achieve. *Samadhi* does not represent 'success' in yoga. It represents the merging of all the collective experiences that arise from the practices of the first seven facets of the Yogic Wisdom, or *yoga darshana,* your way of viewing the world. Your work, dear yogini, is to keep showing up for practice, to keep polishing the facets of your inner jewel, and to remember who you are and want to be in your universe.

Peace and beautiful practice.

Sincerely yours,

Nicole

CHAPTER 13

Wholeheartedly Committed

"If you are willing to be disappointed in your search for the right answer to a problem, for the right thing to do, the right person for the job, just about every situation is a place where an insight might be found."
– Seth Godin

Washington, D.C.—April 6th, 2019

Dear Yogini,

There is something underneath your relationship to yoga that is the actual engine behind your moving forward on your path. It is your commitment, your dedication, the inner resolve you bring to doing the work of yoga that invites you to cultivate a harmonious relationship with yourself. Your yoga practice can be like heading to the safe, empty, and peaceful space of your attic with its old stained-glass window and soft diffuse light. It's your happy place away from the hubbub of the household, away from the fray of life. You've come up to dust the cobwebs, you tell yourself, but really, you love the clarity you feel when you're there.

Then there's that unforeseen moment when your yoga brings you up against the rock and the hard place within yourself, the conflicts and denials entrenched deep in your too-human psyche that have been dismissed and packaged away. It's the cellar space, dark and dank, with its stacks of boxes shoved up against the moist walls. In these boxes are fragments of realities too uncomfortable or disquieting to your younger self to be entirely forgettable, and so they take up residence in the body, memories frozen in time and space in the subconscious mind. It turns out, the brain doesn't select which files to save and which to delete, so it feels a little unsettling to be on your own in this dark place of uncertainty, on this archeological dig into your past.

As you unpack your boxes in the cellar, the dilemma you have will dredge up your preoccupations and your fears and all the dramas of your own making—we all have them. Your yoga practice then is to bear witness to the conditioned patterns of reactivity that show up in the fleeting empty space between stimulus and response. Little by little, your practice—reflected in your body, your emotions, your thoughts and inner dialogue—will reveal to you the ways in which your well-trained amygdala screams at you, *Resist! Run! Hide!* And in the space of noticing this tightening or closing down to your experience, you might breathe instead and choose then to be with your tendencies without indulging them.

You access the attic with ease because it offers you a pleasurable experience. The door to the cellar on the other hand is old, heavy, and slightly rotted in places. It's a bugger to move. Opening this door is the commitment you are willing to make to do the work of clearing out the boxes and cleaning up the cellar. It's the inner resolve you bring to being with yourself, especially when it feels difficult, like when you feel isolated and alone, sad or angry, afraid or just not brave. You will sit with all the boxes around you, and one by one, breath by breath, practice by practice, you will begin the arduous task of unpacking them.

Yoga, in the practice of *asana*, has nothing to do with what you can or cannot do physically. Being truly strong and resilient has much more to do with how willing you are to look at yourself, the resolve you bring to being with what shows up in your practice, and how well you learn to open your heart, how well you learn to let go and let be. It is conceivable that *avidya*, ignorance, is bliss, but the ego will always be self-limiting by virtue of its manipulations to enhance its sense of 'I-am-ness' (*asmita*), its tendencies towards pleasure-seeking (*raga*) and its opposite, pain-avoidance (*dvesha*), and ultimately the fear of death (*abhinivesha*).

These five afflictions, or *kleshas* in the Yogic Wisdom (*sutra II.3*) describe what it means to be human and subject to the human condition. As the ego continues to indulge ignorance (*avidya*), you cannot help but then be limited in your experiences of the world. Too much pride in your accomplishments, say your achievement of a particular *asana*, will diminish your experience of joy in the pose. It'll cause you to envy another's perceived successes in yoga, to focus all your energy and attention to what you think and believe you lack, and to look upon another yogin with negative regard. To view your own endeavors as negative will categorically suck you dry.

The alchemical process of yoga requires of you a willingness to step into the 'cellar' of your practice and into the shadows of your ego-self and, from this place of disquiet or discontent, dedicate yourself to the practice of all yogic principles, from *yama* to *dhyana*. You then develop the tenacity to be present with the enemies of the heart (your envy, anger, pride, greed, attachments and lust) and with the many impediments to practice. Your practice acts upon imperfection and resistance to show you your singular humanity. Your commitment to step into your shadow aspects and experience your humanness requires a degree of vulnerability, a readiness to be with the emotional sensitivities of the heart. To be present with every fiber of your being is the catalyst to trusting yourself and thus holding safe space for the whole of your being.

Be truthful in the ways you show up for yourself on your mat and on your cushion. And be patient on this path of discovery and growth. Over time and with practice, you learn to trust the process of yoga and come to understand that nothing—not your fears, not your anger, not your past hurts, not your secret desires—can take away your sincerity of heart. This dedication to showing up regardless and to believing without any tendril of doubt in the fundamental truth of your self-worth and basic goodness is what Patañjali calls *mahavrtam,* or 'heart vow'.

Mahavrtam will support the task at hand as you work with your yoga to navigate the impediments which obstruct your progress and distract your mind. There are three kinds of *città,* or mindsets, according to Patañjali: those that are self-inflicted (through false thinking or 'wrong cognition'); those caused by imbalances in the body; and problems brought about by the circumstances of life. While many twists of fate in life can feel out of your control, you do have control over the content and quality of your thoughts.

Billions of thoughts arise insistent and unbidden all day long (and sometimes all night too). They float in the air like particles of dust, invisible until they land on something solid. Under the right circumstances—when you are paying attention to the games your mind plays—your thoughts too can land in the sphere of your consciousness and become something tangible that you can perceive with your senses. You will find yourself with a limitless supply of thoughts to choose from by constant, virtual connection to this thinking realm!

The key here is that, in practice, your consciousness gets to sift through your thoughts and choose the right thoughts for you; dust off the ones that do not want to deal with right now. Problems show up when the stickier thoughts (conditioned or habitual), the ones that aren't filtered out, keep circulating in your mind over and over again, then nag and shift your physical and energetic-emotional dynamic in negative ways. These stickier thoughts become thought forms and manifest in the physiology as physical and mental imbalances in the form of dis-ease and symptomatology.

Thought forms can feel impossible to challenge. The more you fight them, the more you think about it, and the more resistance seems to build. What you're saying to yourself is, "I am going to fix this" or "I am not going to think about this" or "this needs to be something other than it is;" The only thing these thought forms do is create more of 'this' in your body; so instead of getting rid of these thoughts, you will find that you are energizing them even more. So consciously release these thought forms from your consciousness each time they show; allow them to "dissolve" rather than take up residence in the hallways of your mind.

We do not always have control over the nature of our thoughts, but once we are aware of them, we can consciously shift their dynamic to serve in our favor. What I have discovered for myself is that the thoughts that overwhelm me the most are more often than not related to narratives that belong to some familial, cultural, or societal paradigm that neither belongs to me nor works for me. Somewhere along my merry way, I appropriated entire storylines that dictated my thoughts, then my feelings, and then the way I was in the world and how I manifested that in my life.

We are trained so well in our culture to fix something perceived as broken (or not perfect enough), to manage the unmanageable, and control outcome according to a certain idea or plan of what that looks like. The problem is most of the time this modus operandi engenders something akin to resistance. I'm sure you have had the experience of trying to access a posture in yoga practice that feels out of reach. Perhaps you have a determination that surmounts all odds (which hopefully does not leave you with a pulled muscle or tendon); mostly, the harder you try to get into the pose, the more Sisyphean it feels, witnessing over and over your futile attempts.

The key here is not to fight your resistance to what is and not to try to solve the problem with your thinking. Instead, the yoga asks you to perceive the resistance, to bring consciousness to its presentation in your body, in your mind, in your soul, and then to switch your focus towards tacit acknowledgement with clear boundaries for yourself as to what is acceptable to you and what is not.

Now, shift the paradigms dictated by your thoughts. New ways of thinking emerge that enable you to engage in actions that work in your service. Thereby you invite a different outcome from the one you originally forecast or imagined on the basis of false premises, assumptions, and expectations. Once you realize that you have control over the content of your thoughts, it is inevitable that your life will reflect this back to you from the outside; essentially your power goes where you mind goes. Conversely, when resistance arises—and it will—take note, and come back to your practice of choosing the focus of your thinking and the nature of your intention and then send them in the direction you wish them to go.

The Yogic Wisdom offers you a way to navigate the impediments and the conflicts that arise as a condition of life and living. Befriend each and every obstacle you encounter in practice and in life, if only for the purpose of meeting yourself at the heart of your dilemma so you might then live into your own unique answer. *To be or not to be a yoga teacher?*

The inevitable shift of awareness and consciousness that comes up as a side-effect of your practice, intentionally and unintentionally, will be met with sometimes impossible circumstances, unimaginable obstacles, and always the unpredictability and inevitability of life and of being human. Use the teachings of yoga as the substrate of your own practice to determine your path. And assume responsibility for walking this path in your truth. Just as the natural largesse of life is filled with pettiness and prejudices and violence and greed—all expressions of the ignorance that lies beneath—so too is the yoga industry replete with its own contradictions and capitalistic tendencies, plagued by the ubiquitous sense of "me, myself, and I" that drives success-oriented and power-driven sensitivities.

The yoga profession, while loosely moderated by the general certifying body known as the Yoga Alliance (26), is not subject to external oversight, which means that schools of yoga and yoga teachers alike set their own standards of excellence. You will need to practice all the yogic principles (*yama, niyama, asana, pranayama, pratyahara, dharana* and *dhyana*), embrace the moral, ethical, physical, mental, intellectual, and spiritual disciplines of yoga, and above all, listen in upon your heart or soul's calling. *How can your yoga best serve you and in what capacity?*

What shows up on your yoga mat is reflective of how you live your life and perhaps too what needs to shift. Maybe your yoga has changed your perspective on things. Maybe you are feeling the positive effects of your practice in the sphere of your life too. Maybe you think you want to become a yoga teacher. But what if becoming a yoga teacher is not the point but rather the potential side-effect of your journey? Why shortchange yourself on any experience, positive or negative, by deciding ahead of time what the outcome is going to be?

This is the point that the very teachings of the *Bhagavad Gita* make. This 'Song of the Spirit' stands on its own merit as an epic poem in the large body of ancient Indian texts, and tells us to act from a place of selfless service and to not get attached to the fruits of our labors. Whether you decide to become a yoga teacher or not, be a yoga practitioner for the sake of being a yoga practitioner. If you apply yourself wholeheartedly to your craft, then the path will unfold before you from a place of trust and sincerity within yourself.

And you should ask nothing less of any teacher in whom you choose to place your trust. They must understand their own shortcomings and embody the qualities you wish to cultivate for yourself on and off the mat. Use your yoga and touch in upon your heart to discern which teacher or teachers of yoga most honestly serve your intentions and best interests. There are those who will wittingly and unwittingly present themselves as enlightened gurus, or healers, or who will sell you something you don't really want—any profession is prey to such quackery. On the flipside of the coin, there are students who will buy into whatever is being sold without a full understanding of what it is exactly they have subscribed to. (27)

So practice discernment. No one is going to hand you enlightenment on a silver platter, although they may well try. Figure out what you want. Know what you need. Decide how far you are willing to go and how much you are willing to commit in time and dollars and energy to get it. And finally, who do you trust and are they aligned with you?

Deep within each of us is a seat of sacredness that cannot be defiled by any action because we are grace and we are beauty and we are brilliance and we are love. But I know too from personal experience how susceptible we are to believing the narratives that our doubt or our insecurities or our immutable principles and paradigms tell us. It is second nature to become attached in some way to some principled idea or emotion or place or person, and then that has the potential to become the focal point for our energies.

You will come to understand if you have not yet, that resolution of your inner conflict can only come by acknowledging that conflicting truths can and do exist: That you can want to be a yoga teacher in one respect and not want to be a yoga teacher in another; that your yoga practice doesn't just happen on the mat or in a studio. You can take this practice of curiosity and non-judgment and a heightened quality of consciousness into your life and the way you want to be in the world in accordance with your own truth. And you don't have to try to change who you are—that's just adding resistance—but become *more* of who you already are, and let yourself soar. Keep showing up for your yoga with the integrity and the grit and all the perfect imperfections that make you You.

Maybe it is that you stand at a crossing of the ages, dear yogini, where you cannot remain standing in these divisions-in-motion. Step onto your path, away from any sense of disconnect from yourself or the dejection that undermines your best efforts. Beware of those who distort the yogic wisdom to meet perceived needs or outer goals, or your own inclinations to reconcile yourself with the ignorance of the world. Absorb your own destiny and transform it within yourself by living it forward through your practice of yoga.

As you persist along this path of yoga, make three resolutions to reduce the all-pervasive *abhinivesha,* fear of death, also the fear of living life to its fullest: First, get to know yourself through yoga and meditation, and live your vision of an honest and selfless life. Second, open your heart to sincere and unconditional love, of yourself and others. Third, live your "one wild and precious life" (28) in the image of your truth so you have no regrets.

May your beautiful path unfold before you.

I am a reflection of you, and you of me, in our common humanity.

Namastē,

Nicole

CLOSING

Jai!

"When you are inspired by some great purpose, some extraordinary project, all your thoughts break their bounds. Your mind transcends limitations, your consciousness expands in every direction and you find yourself in a new, great and wonderful world. Dormant forces, faculties and talents become alive and you discover yourself to be a greater person by far than you ever dreamed yourself to be."
— **Patañjali**

Winchester, MA—May 1ˢᵗ, 2019

Dear Yogini,

Let us be human together and speak of our disappointments, our grief, sometimes our fear, but also of our courage and our trust regarding all things that yoga brings to life. Please know I hold and honor your confidences and your sentiments in the highest esteem because they are each and every one of them valid and very, very real, and I have experienced every single one in my own fashion. Faced with various conflicting truths along your path, you will need to consider the urge to move forward—a movement into uncertainty—and the urge to resist, to hold onto what feels certain and what you think you know and want to control. Change is hard under the best of circumstances; under hardship or duress, it may feel impossible. You will face the need to let go because there is nothing left for you to hold onto; and the desire to hold on because it feels impossible to let go.

To live in truth, as it turns out, is to be able to live in these contradictions, to accept that each element can be true without negating the other. When your heart grows so big it can contain the right and the wrong, the good and the bad, the happy and the sad, your courage and your fears, know that your yoga is working in service of *you*. I know this because I too am practicing living with all the contradictions life has placed at my own feet in what feels like too small a heart to contain all of these sensitivities: The grief of loss mixed up with the joys of celebration; the intimacy of family transmuting into the independence of empty-nest; the known of a yoga studio relinquished for the unknown of self-agency; the complexities of couplehood dissolving into the simplicity of singledom; from Here to another Now.

What lessons can you derive from your experiences on the mat to revitalize your expression of yourself off the mat and in your life? What does your calling to seek more from your yoga feel like in your body? What does it sound like in your heart? Your yoga reveals to you your particular gift. Find your voice, your self-expression and shout to the world what you are about. As you persevere at the practice of the Yogic Wisdom and in following your path of yoga, you will find that signs and motivations show up in your sphere of awareness in the most mundane and also unlikely places, from your coffee mug to a pop-up ad on Facebook. Simply take notice, this is all that yoga asks of you.

You do not need to be an expert at yoga, dear yogini; you will become the expert of your own experiences by your engagement with the tenets and practices of the Yogic Wisdom and your wholehearted commitment to your path. *Adhikara* is a Sanskrit term that implies openness to deeper spiritual study combined with a respect for what is being studied. It also suggests ownership in that every student assumes a certain level of responsibility for their yoga and what they do with it, commensurate with their body of knowledge and degree of commitment to their practice. So I reflect your question back to you, dear yogini, and ask you instead: *In what capacity do you perceive your experiences, through yoga and your "inmost happening," working to serve your highest truth?* You have within you all the resources you need to meet yourself fully whether that means continuing down the path of yoga in studentship, as a guide, or in some other creative capacity as a "dispeller of darkness." To bring the essence of You into Action in the world is teaching yoga.

Take what you learn off the mat into your daily life. Combine your solitary practices with nature where true healing is found. Carve out time and space for yourself, for self-practice, and for ritual wellbeing. This is a statement of self-worth. You are deserving of everything you want for yourself, and I would be happy to support you on your journey should the need arise. In the end, we are a mandala of practitioners—students, guides, and gurus—who come together through yoga to practice and learn from each other. We feel what it is to breathe, to appreciate the gift of the physical body, the joy of movement, and to experience moments of stillness and equanimity within ourselves, transporting all of this into community and connection. The doorway to practice is always open and the path of Self-mastery is constantly evolving.

Little do I know of you or your life, but I do know this from my heart: You are as brilliant as the stars, as vast as the skies, and as temperamental and troubled as the seas, for you are a child of the universe and subject too to the mere fact of being human. Let amazement, furious curiosity, and passionate perseverance fuel your thirst for all things bright and beautiful, for you are a Seeker—this I know to be true. Light up your world with trust and truth and love and, together, in connection, let us learn to trust the untrustworthy and be brave.

Embody your truth and love yourself without condition. Ultimately, the place of practice is your very own heart, this place of conscious intent. The one thing we all have in common is our humanity. On some level each of us participates in our own 'hero's journey' to remember who we are, what we are, and where we are on this path of life. What makes yoga such a powerful practice is that it asks us to step right into seeing the habitual and conceptual conditioning of our consciousness into the freedom of begin fresh, and merely human, for a time, together. Anything less is 'spiritual bypass'. The way you live your life—the speed, noise, chaos, agendas, calcifications and conflicts—will all show up on your mat. Take notice. Shift this dynamic for yourself in practice for **NOW** is the time to take this precious yoga out into our lives, our relationships and into the world as a manifestation of the consciousness we cultivate on our individual mats. Join me in taking this heart vow: "*I do.*"

May all be well with mankind.

May the leaders of this Earth protect in every way by keeping to the right path.

May there be goodness for those who know the Earth to be sacred.

May all beings everywhere know peace.

May the rains fall on time and the Earth yield her fruit in abundance.

May this world be free from disturbances, and the righteous free from fear.

Om Shanthi. Shanthi. Shanthi.

> **– Closing Ashtanga Incantation**

Love,

Nicole

Acknowledgements

I have compiled these letters on yoga for the Yogini, the female practitioner of yoga specifically because She is who I know best. I worked with the yoga darshana of Patañjali to frame what I have come to learn of yoga, of myself and of my life through yoga. With the yogic teachings, I illuminate one of many footpaths to living your brightest Self. My hope is that these letters will motivate you to dig deep into your own valient efforts and inspire the manner in which you show up for yourself in practice. May you remain curious about and friendly towards the stuff that rises to the surface and extend this inquisitiveness and kindness to yourself in yoga, to your relationships off the mat, and then into the world at large. *"Be the change you wish to see in the world,"* Mahatma Gandhi reminds me every morning as I savor my coffee from its inspired container.

I extend a dedication and a huge debt of gratitude to *You*, my student, yogin extraordinaire. You have shown up through thick and thin—job loss, divorce, parents to care for, lives to save, kids to feed, cases to plead… I am grateful you came to your practice with your joys and your sorrows as I came with mine. It is no easy task to be with the most vulnerable parts of ourselves on our yoga mat, and I honor that always. Greet your practice every day in some respect or another and be good to yourself. And be kind to new teachers—they are going way out on a limb. May we continue to walk this path together with humility, in connection, and in community.

Thank you to my teachers: Nancy Gilgoff in the Ashtanga vinyasa lineage of Sri K. Patthabi Jois, for validating and trusting me in my teaching, for giving me the tools of touch and an understanding of kinesthetic and energetic awareness; to Zoë Stewart in the lineage of B.K.S. Iyengar who taught me everything I know about feeling inside of myself—your gift of words to evoke physical sensitivity and inner discernment completely shifted my practice and understanding of yoga and allowed me to touch the grief around my father's death and the demise of my marriage by feeling into qualities of the heart I had no idea how to access; to Reverend Gita Beth Bryant, Reiki Master Teacher extraordinaire, you are one of the most knowledgeable people I know in the teachings of yoga—I imbibe every single teaching you transmit, and thank you for the devotion you bring to these teachings; to Kenji, in whose presence I was and could be entirely me, for better and for worse; to my former husband, the father of my children, what can I say? You are my greatest teacher, for no one has shown me more clearly to myself than you.

To Angela Lauria and her fantastic team, thank you for kicking my butt into action; and to my editor, Todd Hunter, for bringing this manuscript into manifestation. I have learned so much from everyone, most importantly, that anything is possible. Thank you, All, for helping me cross "write a book" off my bucket list! And finally, a big thank you to David Hancock and the Morgan James Publishing team for helping me bring this book to print.

To my Mother: Thank you for being a constant in my life and for teaching me to believe in family even when it changes shape and for demonstrating what being a resilient woman looks like. You rock!

To my Father: I love you. I miss you every day still and thank you for your persistent and somewhat sardonic posthumous presence in my life—you do not for a moment let me forget to behave well in the world or make precious space for myself, even if it means parking a ladder in my path plus two black eyes later for me to catch your drift!

To my Soul Sisters and Devoted Yoginis: Christina, Wendy, Lara, Lena, Janet, Maureen, Marilyn, Carolyn, Cecile, Christine, Connie, Cynthia, Dorothy, Genevieve, Sue J, Yan, and so many more! I count myself lucky to have the kinds of friends with whom I can share confidences and cares, and be my most untoward self and still find myself on the receiving end of their benevolence and friendship and love.

Thank you, Mary Corlett—may you rest in peace, beloved friend and guide—for reminding me of my Mother Bear.

And finally, to Claudia and to Mark: Thank you for choosing me to be your mother and for teaching me to love large. From where I stand, I have struck gold. The sole conditions I have for myself with regards to you are to keep you safe, to listen to you, and to love you. My sole intention is to continue to emulate for you, as my father did for me, equal parts independence and how to be in the world—kind, generous, good, fearless, and forces to be reckoned with. Whether I can take any credit for any part of who you each are and the fearlessness with which you both engage your respective lives, know this: I stand in such admiration of you, Mark, and you, Claudia, and love you both to the moon and back.

With all my love and deepest gratitude for all the gifts of grace and blessings all of you have shared.

Love,

Nicole

Notes

1. I discovered a less dogmatic translation and commentary of *The Yoga Sutras, The Yoga Darshana,* by John Wells, which quite spoke to me and my experience of the Yogic Wisdom, at http://darshanapress.com/The%20Yoga%20Darshana.pdf

2. Sankalpa typically translates as 'intention' or 'intentionality' or 'inner resolution.'

3. From Samadhi: *The Highest State of Wisdom: Yoga the Sacred Science,* by Swami Rama, Himalayan Institute Hospital Trust, 2002

4. This unique interpretation of yama and niyama is derived from Nischala Joy Devi's distinctive *Woman's Guide to the Heart and Spirit of the Yoga Sutras, The Secret Power of Yoga,* Three Rivers Press, NY, 2007; pp.177 and 205

5. In Barbara Stoler Miller's translation of *The Yoga Sutra Attributed to Patañjali, YOGA: Discipline of Freedom,* Bantam Books, 1988, p.40

6. Amongst them, John Wells, in http://darshanapress.com/ The%20Yoga%20Darshana.pdf

7. In his translation and annotation of *The Yoga Sūtras of Patañjali* (originally published by Harvard University Press, Cambridge, MA, 1927) Dover edition, unabridged republication, 2003.

8. John Wells, *The Yoga Darshana*, http://darshanapress.com/ The%20Yoga%20Darshana.pdf, p.7.

9. Translation of sutra I.28 by James Haughton Woods in *The Yoga Sūtras of Patañjali* (originally published by Harvard University Press, Cambridge, MA, 1927) Dover edition, unabridged republication, 2003.

10. Nischala Joy Devi's quoted definitions of Yama and Niyama from her book *The Secret Power of Yoga*, Three Rivers Press, NY, 2007, lend a definitive female voice to a discipline that, while formulated during the Sat Yuga, or Golden Age of Indo-Aryan Civilization, is very much grounded in male perspective.

11. Deborah Adele, *Yamas & Niyamas: Exploring Yoga's Ethical Practice,* On-Word Bound Books, Minnesota, 2009

12. According to "The 2016 Yoga in America Study" conducted by Yoga Journal and Yoga Alliance.

13. Translation by James Haughton Woods, *The Yoga Sutras of Patañjali*, Dover Edition, 2003.

14. As my brother, Eric Grant, relates in his book chronicling my father's mysterious and amazing life in *Peregrinations, A Man's Journey,* Writer's Club Press, iUniverse, Inc.2003 (p.71).

15. Abhyasa and vairagya are introduced by Patañjali in YS. I.12 and can be compared to the two wings of a bird to illuminate that abhyasa—which implies action without interruption—and vairagya—which signifies an 'un-coloring' of our consciousness from the things we get attached to—work together to bring the mind to a place of stillness.

16. My favorite translation of this sutra (that I have come across in my study of yoga) comes from BKS Iyengar's translation in *Light on the Yoga Sūtras of Patañjali*, Thorson's Harper Collins, 1996, p. 149.

17. This is the knowledge substantiated by the fairly recent field of research known as neuroplasticity—the capacity of the human brain (like muscles) to reorganize itself by forming new neural connections throughout life, and to adjust their activities in response to new situations or to changes in their environment; in essence, for the brain to repattern with repetition and frequency over time. This has fundamental implications for validating yoga as a science as well as a philosophy and practice, and increases our understanding of how bringing the mind into more and more discerning and intentional ways of moving the body in asana can help us shift mindsets as well as ways of framing and perceiving ourselves and the world around us.

18. The vagus nerve is the tenth cranial nerve and interfaces with parasympathetic control (also known as rest and relaxation response) of the heart, lungs, and digestive tract. It extends all the way from the brainstem down through the chest to beyond the stomach and also carries sensory information from the internal organs back to the brain. The ventral vagal complex is our Social Engagement System (located above the diaphragm it regulates facial cues, tone, language, etc.) and the dorsal vagal complex is our Passive Defense System (located below the diaphragm it regulates immobilization, freeze and collapse response). When the nervous system is dysregulated over and over again (low vagal tone) it takes very little to trigger an over-reactive (or post-traumatic) response. More and more research suggests that a healthy vagus nerve is vital to our ability to attune to others (empathy), to see and be seen emotionally (social bonding) and

to feel safe, which is why yoga is such a powerful modality in healing as it serves to increase vagal tone and thus increase our window of tolerance and resilience to stressful and/or traumatic situations.

19. In sutra II.28 of *The Yoga Sūtras*.

20. From *Saint Francis and the Sow* by Galway Kinnell, Three Books. Copyright © 2002 by Galway Kinnell.

21. In sutra II.19 Patañjali analyzes nature (prakriti) by identifying the progressive layers of its manifestation in the mind.

22. Sūtra I.2 - *yogaś-citta-vṛtti-nirodhaḥ* is Patañjali's definition of Yoga.

23. Nischala Joy Devi's translation of yoga sutra I.41 in *The Secret Power of Yoga*, Three Rivers Press, NY, 2007. pp. 90

24. Sutra I.41 in BKS Iyengar's translation in *Light on the Yoga Sūtras of Patañjali*, Thorsons, Harper Collins Pub. 1993, p. 87.

25. In Barbara Stoler Miller's translation of the yoga sutra attributed to Patañjali, *YOGA: Discipline of Freedom*, Bantam Books, 1988, p.40.

26. The Yoga Alliance (www.yogaalliance.org) is an American-based agency and largest nonprofit association representing the yoga community at large.

27. An example of this is seen in the recent *New York Times* article, "Should Every American Citizen Be a Yoga Teacher? CorePower, the country's largest yoga studio chain, is leading the way," Alice Hines, April 6, 2019.

28. From Mary Oliver's poem, *The Summer Day*, "House of Light," Beacon Press, 1990.

Thank You

In Yogini's Dilemma, I explore how the yoga practitioner can step into the heart of her conflict (any conflict) using the methodology of yoga to inform her life and walk the path of being true to herself, as a teacher of yoga or not. I address the female yoga practitioner for the simple reason this is the experience I entertain in this life, but I hope all yoga practitioners alike will feel some relevance in aspects of this book and find some practical nuggets of wisdom within.

I invite you to view my video book bonus, accessible through my website at www.yogamandala.com/bookbonus, in which I offer you, the practitioner of yoga, strategies for how to M.A.P (motivate, authenticate & potentiate) Your Yoga™ and bring it to life on and off the mat. Email me at nicole@yogamandala.com to receive your free 40-minute chakra yoga video practice based on the eight limbs of yoga or set up a free 15-minute strategy session.

Namastē

Nicole

About the Author

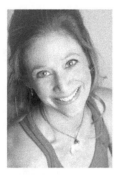

Nicole A. Grant is a certified yoga therapist, author and personal & professional transformational strategist who brings over two decades of dedicated yoga practice and experiential research in the lineage of Sri T. Krishnamacharya to her visionary programs and unique style of teaching. The practice of tuning 'in', embodying with wisdom, and seeing clearly the stories we create or tell ourselves in our mind is the basis for restructuring the personal and professional belief systems that undermine integrity and positive outcomes in work, family and life.

Yoga Mandala was founded in 2001 with the purpose of making yoga accessible to everyone from all walks of life. The academy is geared to practitioners of yoga who seek to 'do more' with their yoga, where the question becomes not so much whether to be a yoga teacher or not, but rather, how to bring one's yoga to life and extend one's yoga into action in the world. Yoga Mandala Academy's innovative self-mastery & marketing intensives and strategic leadership training & certification programs are founded in the proven power of yoga methodology and source the yoga practitioner's skill sets to leverage their yoga in all aspects of life. Be a part of the Yoga Mandala mission to motivate, authenticate and potentiate your yoga in the world.

Learn more about Nicole on *Boston Voyager* (http://bostonvoyager.com/interview/meet-nicole-grant-yoga-mandala-winchester-ma-north-boston/).

Connect with Nicole at:

www.yogamandala.com

https://www.facebook.com/YogaMandalaAcademy/

https://www.instagram.com/yoloyogini/

CPSIA information can be obtained
at www.ICGtesting.com
Printed in the USA
LVHW111822270420
654541LV00008B/1702

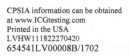

9 781642 797749